THE
DAIRY-FREE
KETO
DIET COOKBOOK

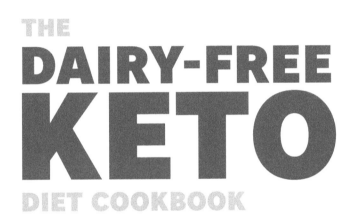

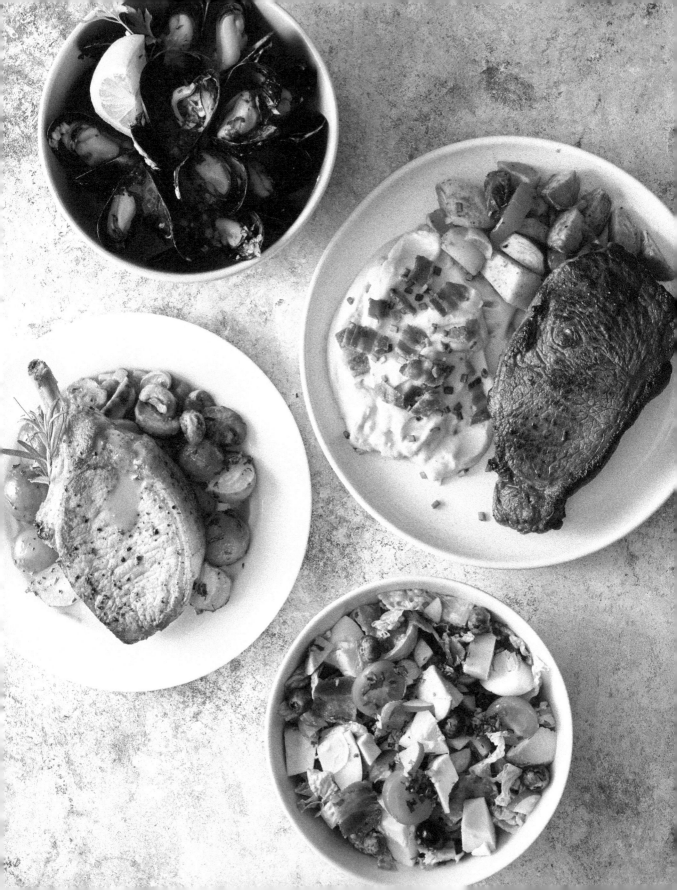

THE DAIRY-FREE KETO

DIET COOKBOOK

SATISFYING HIGH-FAT RECIPES TO FUEL YOUR HEALTH

Jessica Dukes

Photography by Darren Muir

ROCKRIDGE
PRESS

For general information on our other products and services or to obtain technical support, please contact our Customer Care Department within the U.S. at (866) 744-2665, or outside the U.S. at (510) 253-0500.

Rockridge Press publishes its books in a variety of electronic and print formats. Some content that appears in print may not be available in electronic books, and vice versa.

Cover Design: Suzanne LaGasa
Interior Design: Debbie Berne
Editor: Bridget Fitzgerald
Production Editor: Andrew Yackira
Photography: Darren Muir
Food Styling: Yolanda Muir

ISBN: Print 978-1-64152-278-6 | eBook 978-1-64152-279-3

To my dad who taught me to love,
my mom who taught me to serve,
and Brad who taught me to shine.

Keto Faux Cappuccino, page 26

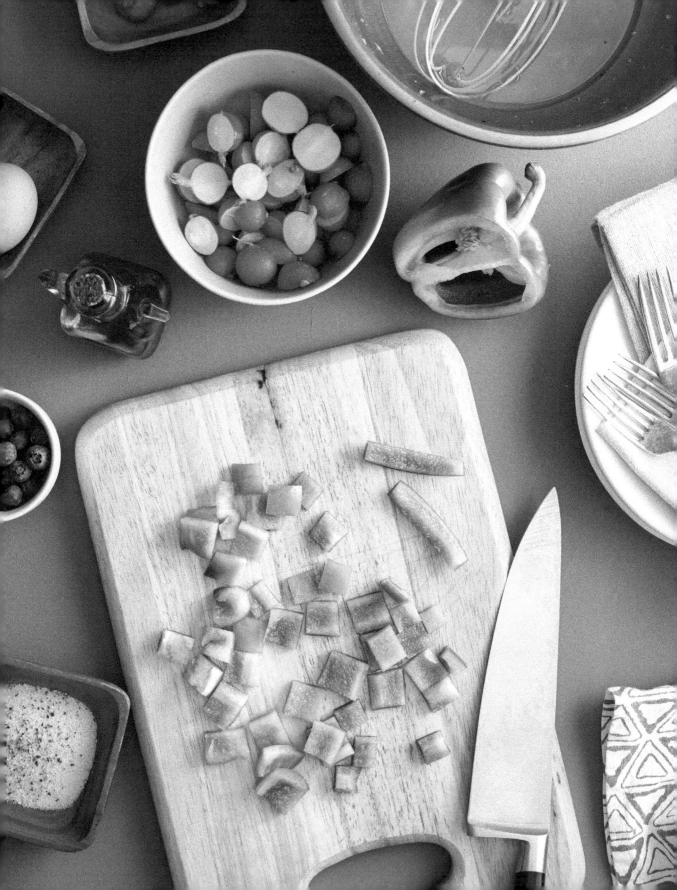

CONTENTS

INTRODUCTION

Not so long ago, I needed a change.

I had been happily married for almost five years and was feeling very lucky in love, but at the same time, I had spent all five of those years struggling with health and body issues. I was chasing fad diets trying to lose weight, only to gain it all back when those unsustainable diets became, well, unsustainable. I had been diagnosed with polycystic ovary syndrome (PCOS) 10 years before, and I was trying desperately to find the right dietary or lifestyle change to aid with the symptoms. Health was and had always been my ultimate goal, but I was feeling exhausted and hopeless.

I will never forget that December night when I found the solution—though I didn't know it yet. I was sitting on the couch, frustrated with how I was feeling and with my overall health. Not knowing what else to do, I took to Google, and ended up finding an unexpected Internet thread. What I read that night started the process of changing my life in ways I could not have foreseen.

What I came across were the words "ketogenic diet." I had never heard of this way of eating before, and I was intrigued to learn that you could eat all the cheese and all the fat but still lose weight. *Sign me up!* I thought. And as I continued my research, I found article after article stating that PCOS symptoms could be improved by the ketogenic diet. Right then and there, I decided to dive in head-first and try this thing out.

After a few months of eating on the ketogenic diet, I noticed that I had more energy and mental clarity, and my body felt better overall. For the first time in a long time, I wanted to work out. I was losing weight that I needed to lose, and I was even able to stop taking medication for my PCOS symptoms. Because the keto diet was satisfying and easy to incorporate into my everyday life, I realized I could maintain it forever—it was no longer a "diet" for me. Before I knew it, I was gaining confidence.

There was just one problem. After about a year and a half on the keto diet, I began noticing that dairy was causing some issues that I needed to address. I started an elimination diet, removing all dairy, and—shockingly at the time—I dropped 10 pounds in two weeks. I sought out a medical professional, who confirmed my suspicions: Dairy was the major obstacle to my health goals, and a likely cause of inflammation, bloating, and gut issues. But my understanding was that the keto diet—my new lifestyle—relied heavily on dairy for its healthy-fats component.

I considered giving up the keto diet entirely and just going dairy-free instead, but I loved the benefits of the keto diet that I had already implemented. I knew that keto was the way I wanted to eat forever and quickly learned that going dairy-free while eating keto was still doable. There is a way to get in your healthy fats and achieve ketosis (see page 3) without the dairy. All you doubters—I was one of you—keep reading.

Going dairy-free while still maintaining a keto diet can be challenging, it's true. That's why I've written this book—to guide you through and make it as easy as possible, whether you're doing it because of a health need or because you simply prefer dairy alternatives. In the pages that follow, we're headed to my kitchen, where I'll give you easy dairy-free meals without all the fuss. The ingredients can be found at your local grocery store, and most of the meals in this book can be on the table in 30 minutes. What you'll find here are satisfying meals with familiar flavors that you'll want to make over and over. Plus, your entire family—keto or not—will love them.

I can truly say that keto has changed my life and my health, and that dairy-free keto changed everything: It helped me alter my gut health in a permanent way, so that I finally feel good on a regular basis.

It's not only doable—it's easy. From my kitchen to yours, let's dig in and get cooking!

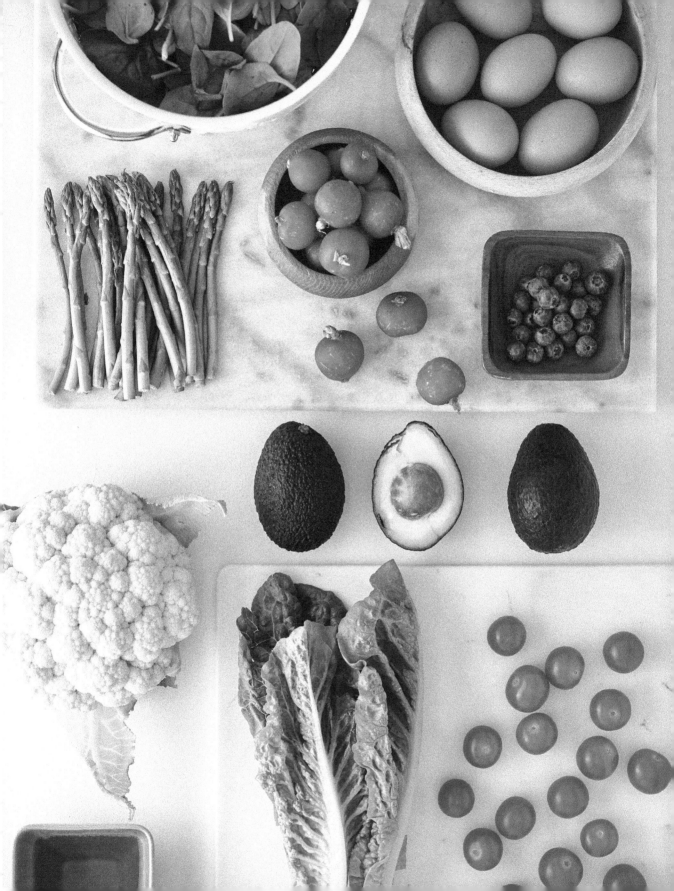

CHAPTER 1

the basics of a dairy-free keto diet

I'm not going to lie—when my suspicion that I needed to go dairy-free was confirmed, I was bummed. Because, obviously, cheese is delicious! But I knew that my health was more important, so I was determined to come up with recipes that would be just as good without the dairy. My husband, Brad, can eat dairy, and I truly don't think he's noticed the sudden lack of cheese in our food, because I've learned to be creative and to use spices to my advantage.

Learning to eat dairy-free on a keto diet can be a little complicated at first, because it goes against everything you learn when becoming a student of keto. Cheese and butter are staples in most ketogenic diets. Add in the dairy-free element, and many people say, "There's no way I can do that!" Yes, you can. In this chapter, we'll cover all the basics you need to get started eating dairy-free keto. And whether you're eating dairy-free because of allergies, gut health, or just a preference, this is the book for you.

I'll teach you how to get enough healthy fats in your body without dairy, how your coffee can still be amazing without cream, and how swapping out butter for good oils is easy and worth it.

How the Ketogenic Diet Works

Simply put, the ketogenic diet is a high-fat, moderate-protein, low-carbohydrate way of eating. Those three macronutrients (or "macros")—fat, protein, and carbs—are the building blocks of all food, and your body needs them to live. Normally, your body uses carbohydrates for energy, but if there aren't enough carbohydrates, it starts using fat instead. This fat-burning metabolic state is known as "ketosis," and to keep it going over the long term, you have to minimize carbs (so your body doesn't switch back to relying on them) and maximize fat (so your body still gets all the energy it needs).

There are plenty of schools of thought on the best way to eat keto, and the correct macronutrient ratio will vary from person to person, but most people are aiming for somewhere in the vicinity of getting 60 to 75 percent of their daily calories from fat, 20 to 30 percent from protein, and 5 to 10 percent from carbs. That said, you'll notice that not every recipe in this book exactly conforms to that ratio. This is to allow you to combine different recipes so that your overall intake for the day falls within the percentages. Use this flexibility to balance various recipes—maybe something higher in carbs for breakfast, and much lower for dinner—in order to structure your day of eating around the most effective ratio for you. Some people count macros religiously, while others have become experienced enough with the keto diet to correctly estimate which foods will add up to the right daily macro balance for their body. Either way, macros are your starting point. You won't learn how to eat ketogenically if you don't know the macro ratios your body needs to get and stay in ketosis.

So the first thing you want to do when starting a keto diet is find a reliable keto macro calculator (I like the one available at ruled.me). This will help you determine what ratio of carbs, fat, and protein you need for your own specific body to get into ketosis. And you can go from there.

Because I've eaten within the ketogenic diet for two and a half years, I don't count my macros much anymore. I'm pretty schooled in what I can and can't eat, so I just keep a loose tally in my head. But I started off counting my macros carefully, and occasionally, if I feel like my body is off or if my weight goals have changed substantially, I go back to it. Whether you're writing your counts in a journal, keeping them in an app, or tallying them in your head, always know what you're fueling your body with at all times. That's the key.

The Benefits of Dairy-Free Keto

People choose to go dairy-free for a number of reasons. Perhaps the most common is lactose intolerance (the inability to digest lactose, the sugar found in milk)—which 65 percent of people in the world have, according to the National Institutes of Health. There are a host of additional medical conditions and symptoms that can be negatively impacted by dairy consumption, and it's important to check in with your health and assess whether eliminating dairy might help you achieve your specific desires and goals. If you have any of the following conditions, consider whether dairy-free might be the right modifier for your keto diet. It certainly was for me.

STOMACH PAIN: When stomach pain results from food sensitivities, it can be difficult to pinpoint the problem. An elimination diet can be helpful, and often, the problem turns out to be dairy products. In my case, my stomach was often hurting and uneasy, even after I had adapted to the keto diet. Once I went dairy-free, the problem was solved.

SEVERE BLOATING: The inability to break down lactose can lead to major digestive problems, including gas and bloating. For those already prone to inflammation, dairy can aggravate the symptoms.

CONSTIPATION: Many people prone to constipation are sensitive to certain ingredients, dairy being one of them.

GUT HEALTH: The impact of dietary changes on the human microbiome (the trillions of bacteria, viruses, and fungi that make up much of the body) is a constantly expanding area of science. According to the T.H. Chan School of Public Health at Harvard University, certain dietary influences can cause a disturbance in the balance of coexisting microbiota in the body. It wasn't until dairy-free keto helped me heal my gut that I even realized this was the root of so many of my issues.

LACTOSE INTOLERANCE: If you've been holding back from keto because you're lactose intolerant and it seems to involve so much butter and cheese, worry no more! You don't have to eat dairy to eat keto, and you can still reap all the benefits. It's also worth noting that many people are lactose intolerant and don't realize it; in fact, many of the symptoms listed on this page can often be traced back to an absence of lactase, the enzyme that breaks down lactose. If you have even mild issues with certain dairy products, it's something to consider.

WHAT IS THE DIFFERENCE BETWEEN DAIRY-FREE KETO AND PALEO?

The paleo diet is an eating plan based on what prehistoric humans might have eaten. It eliminates grains, legumes, processed sugar, and most dairy sources, but lets you eat meats, eggs, nuts and seeds, fruits, vegetables, unrefined fats and oils, and natural sweeteners (such as maple syrup and honey). Although it is relatively low-carb, it does not restrict carbohydrates to the same degree as the keto diet, and therefore does not engage ketosis.

The keto diet, on the other hand, focuses primarily on the three macronutrients of fat, protein, and carbohydrates. By consuming a lot of fat but not very much protein and very few carbs, someone on the keto diet can induce ketosis, a metabolic state in which the body burns fat instead of carbohydrates for energy.

The big, shiny difference between the two is ketosis—teaching your body to keep burning fat—and that is what we're after.

STALLED WEIGHT LOSS: If you feel like you're doing everything right and still can't get past that stubborn weight-loss plateau, try eliminating dairy. It might just be exactly what your body needs— either because of the conditions named above, such as bloating and lactose intolerance, or simply because it will change your caloric intake.

POLYCYSTIC OVARY SYNDROME (PCOS): According to the U.S. Department of Health and Human Services, PCOS is "one of the most common endocrine disorders among women of reproductive age." Although current studies are inconclusive, it's possible that PCOS symptoms can be aggravated by dairy intake. Further research is needed to draw firm conclusions, but the anecdotal evidence was enough to convince me it was worth a try—and now I can add my own story to that list.

IRRITABLE BOWEL SYNDROME (IBS): Most people with IBS are lactose intolerant, so keeping your diet dairy-free will help alleviate IBS symptoms and aid with stomach comfort.

Setting Yourself Up for Success

We're almost ready to start cooking, but first, let's stock your pantry and refrigerator with dairy-free, keto-friendly ingredients that you'll want to keep on hand to make your meals easier. These essentials on hand will help you resist the urge to reach for convenient but off-limits dairy products when you're hungry.

PANTRY ESSENTIALS

- Almond flour
- Alternative sweeteners, such as Swerve (granulated and confectioners')
- Baking powder
- Bone broth
- Cayenne
- Coconut flour
- Coconut milk, canned
- Coconut, shredded
- Grapeseed oil
- Olive oil
- Pepper, black
- Salt, such as Himalayan pink salt, which is loaded with minerals and trace nutrients; I use it on everything
- Vanilla extract, alcohol-free

REFRIGERATED ESSENTIALS

- Bacon
- Barbecue sauce, sugar-free, low-carb (such as Tessemae's brand)
- Broccoli
- Cauliflower
- Cream cheese, dairy-free (such as Kite Hill brand)
- Eggs
- Ketchup, sugar-free, low-carb (such as Primal Kitchen brand)
- Marinades, sugar-free, low-carb
- Mayonnaise, sugar-free, low-carb (such as Primal Kitchen brand)
- Meats, grass-fed
- Mustard, sugar-free, low-carb (such as Primal Kitchen brand)
- Pickles
- Plain yogurt, dairy-free (such as Kite Hill brand)
- Salami, sugar-free, low-carb
- Other vegetables and greens

OTHER PERISHABLE ESSENTIALS

- Avocados
- Garlic
- Lemons
- Onions
- Tomatoes

THE DEAL WITH GHEE

Many people wonder if ghee, or clarified butter, is the exception to the dairy-free rule. I will not be using ghee throughout this book in order to keep it 100 percent dairy-free, but some people with lactose intolerance are able to tolerate ghee, as it has very low levels of lactose and is thus unlikely to cause a reaction. However, you should always know and understand your own tolerance levels and dietary preferences. For those who can and do use ghee, feel free to replace the oils in my recipes with equal amounts of ghee.

EQUIPMENT

I am a minimalist in the kitchen, and I'm happy to report that the keto diet doesn't require any special equipment or fancy gadgets. With just a few essential pieces of equipment, you'll be able to prepare your food quickly and efficiently, which will make dairy-free keto cooking much more enjoyable.

Must Have

I find myself reaching for these tools more than any others in my kitchen.

CUTTING BOARD: Because you'll be cutting, dicing, and mincing fresh ingredients, you need a proper surface for safe and handy chopping.

CAST IRON SKILLET: I love to cook with a cast iron skillet because it can go straight from stovetop to oven and is an excellent tool for searing and roasting meat. My cast iron skillet was my grandmother's, and every time I use it I think of her (though I'm sure she wasn't cooking keto!).

BLENDER: Because we're creating dairy-free recipes, we lose many of the natural binders that help thicken and hold ingredients together. A blender will help quickly incorporate ingredients.

GOOD KNIFE: A good sharp knife is essential to make all of your ingredients come together (or apart!) more easily. I personally love Cutco-brand knives.

BAKING SHEETS: You can cook everything from salmon to cookies on a baking sheet, so it's great to have two or three 13-by-18-inch rimmed baking sheets on hand. Use nonstick pans or layer parchment paper for easy cleanup.

Nice to Have

Once you've started cooking more often, you might find you'd like a few extra tools to fill out your kitchen arsenal.

STAND MIXER: A stand mixer (rather than a handheld electric mixer) is really nice to have for baking. You can combine your ingredients at the same time as you chop, wash, or perform other kitchen tasks, thereby minimizing your prep time.

BAKING DISHES: I use both 9-by-13-inch and 8-by-11-inch baking dishes a lot when I cook keto meals. Baking dishes have deeper sides than rimmed baking sheets, so they work for a wide range of recipes, from roasts to casseroles to desserts. Enameled cast iron baking sheets are pricey but conduct heat extremely well and are also versatile (they can even be used on the stovetop). Tempered glass (like Pyrex) or enameled ceramic baking dishes are the next best thing; they're durable and most are suitable for use with a wide range of oven temperatures.

MIXING BOWLS: Having small, medium, and large mixing bowls makes cooking so much simpler. They're easy to store and wash, so you'll always have a clean one handy and appropriately sized for your ingredient (which helps avoid messes in the kitchen due to overfilled bowls).

SPLATTER SCREEN: A splatter screen is a game changer for stovetop cooking. You place the screen (usually made of stainless steel or silicone) on top of the active pan to catch any bubbling oils or splashes.

How This Book Makes Dairy-Free Keto Easy

This book is full of fuss-free recipes to make dairy-free keto cooking a delight instead of a hassle, leisurely instead of laborious. Each recipe includes nutritional information and a macro breakdown, so you don't have to do any calculations and can jump right in, depending on your allowances for the day. My goal is for these recipes to help you stay on track, so you're motivated to cook—and therefore eat—dairy-free and keto. To that end, I've tried to make them as simple and straightforward as possible. Look for labels that indicate each recipe's particular utility:

ONE POT These recipes can be made in one vessel. That might be a skillet, sheet pan, baking dish, stovetop pan, or even just a single bowl.

NO COOK These recipes require no cooking at all—perfect for hot summer evenings, super-quick lunches, or just keeping life simple.

30 MINUTES These recipes take under 30 minutes to prepare and cook. Some are even snacks that take under five minutes.

5 INGREDIENTS I've tried to use ingredients you likely already have in your kitchen, and some recipes are so simple they require only five of them (not counting salt, pepper, and oil).

Many recipes also include pointers on how to modify the ingredients, the prep process, or the finished dish. Look for these tips below each recipe:

SIMPLIFY IT! These are time- or energy-saving tips to make the recipe more convenient for busy cooks.

SUBSTITUTION TIP I'll offer swaps for certain ingredients that might not be everyone's favorite, or in order to make the dish suit a variety of dietary needs.

INGREDIENT TIP Look for recipe-prepping shortcuts or additional information on selecting ingredients.

VARIATION TIP Learn how to bring different flavors and textures to a dish.

Top Tips for Success on the Dairy-Free Keto Diet

Below are several tips that will help you as you begin this diet, as well as things to keep in mind as you move toward adapting your favorite recipes to fit within the guidelines of dairy-free keto. As obvious as it might seem, sometimes just leaving out the dairy in a recipe and getting more creative with spices instead is the best option. Use the recipes in this book as inspiration for the kinds of substitutions you can make; my aim is to make meal prep easier so you can establish a sustainable way of eating that will benefit your overall health. Here are a few easy shortcuts to help you along the way.

Use healthy fats for cooking. By replacing butter with good oils like olive, coconut, sunflower seed, and avocado, you can immediately make your recipe dairy-free.

Use dairy-free creamers. Use coconut milk or nut milk (like Nutpods) in place of cream or milk in coffee or tea.

Use nondairy spreads. Use avocado, sugar-free mayonnaise (like Primal Kitchen), or dairy-free cream cheese (like the almond-based cream cheese spread from Kite Hill) in place of butter or cream cheese as a spread.

Use sugar-free mayonnaise in normally dairy-based sauces and dressings. Use sugar-free mayonnaise (like Primal Kitchen) in place of heavy cream, half-and-half, buttermilk, or sour cream in creamy sauces and dressings.

Thicken with coconut or nut milk. Use canned coconut milk or nut milk instead of heavy whipping cream. Use dairy-free cream cheese to thicken sauces and make creamy toppings. You still get the rich, creamy taste, but without any dairy.

Explore vegan cheeses. Some of these are high in carbs, but look for aged vegan cheeses made from nuts and seeds. They're a great substitute when you just have to have that melty, cheesy goodness on your dish.

Just leave off the cheese. It may sound obvious, but the easiest way to make your meals dairy-free is just to skip the cheese. Leave it off burgers, and sprinkle salted nuts or seeds over salads for extra texture and flavor.

Cook in bulk. Big-batch cooking is a super-simple way to minimize effort. It doesn't get easier than reheating delicious leftovers that you made the day before.

Read labels. Diligently read all product labels to ensure that the contents are truly dairy-free. Remember, too, that dairy-free products are often made from high-carb legumes like soy, which means they're not keto friendly. Don't assume that just because it's dairy-free, it's also safe for keto (or vice versa)!

SWAP IT OUT!

Need This?	Use This!
Butter for cooking	Olive oil, avocado oil, coconut oil
Butter for spreading	Avocado, coconut butter
Cream cheese	Dairy-free cream cheese
Greek yogurt	Dairy-free plain yogurt
Heavy cream	Coconut cream (canned)
Cream for coffee	Dairy-free creamers
Milk	Almond milk, cashew milk, coconut milk
Ranch dressing	Avocado oil– or sunflower oil–based dressings (I like Primal Kitchen or Tessemae's)

FOODS TO ENJOY VS. AVOID

enjoy

Meats
- Beef
- Beef liver
- Bison
- Chicken
- Pork
- Seafood
- Sausage (without fillers)
- Turkey

Low-carb veggies
- Asparagus
- Avocados
- Bell peppers
- Broccoli
- Brussels sprouts
- Cabbage
- Cauliflower
- Cucumbers
- Green Beans
- Kale
- Lettuce
- Mushrooms
- Okra
- Olives
- Onions
- Pickles
- Radishes
- Scallions
- Shallots
- Spaghetti squash (in moderation)
- Spinach

Fats
- Almonds
- Avocado oil
- Chia seeds
- Coconut oil
- Flaxseed oil
- Fish oil
- Grapeseed oil
- MCT (medium-chain triglycerides) oil (such as coconut oil)
- Olive oil

in moderation

Nuts & seeds*
- Almonds
- Cashews
- Chia seeds
- Flaxseeds
- Hazelnuts
- Macadamia nuts
- Nut butters
- Peanuts
- Pecans
- Pili nuts
- Pine nuts
- Pistachios
- Pumpkin seeds
- Walnuts

*Nuts can add up to too many extra calories if you aren't careful. Watch your portions here.

Berries
- Blackberries
- Blueberries
- Raspberries
- Strawberries

Artificial sweeteners**
- Erythritol (such as Swerve)
- Monk fruit sweetener
- Stevia

**Low-carb sweeteners can be enjoyed in moderation, as your daily macros allow.

I use Swerve, but if you prefer another option, you can find many online resources that supply appropriate conversions. Please note that though erythritol is technically a carbohydrate, its effect on blood sugar is a net zero; you'll see that every recipe that includes Swerve has been calculated without factoring it into the macros, and instead has a separate listing for the amount of erythritol used.

restrict or avoid

Dairy
- Cheese
- Cream
- Cream cheese
- Milk
- Yogurt

Carbs
- Breads
- Candy
- Corn
- Pasta
- Potatoes
- Rice
- Winter squashes

Fruits (other than berries)
- Apples
- Apricots
- Bananas
- Dates
- Grapefruit
- Grapes
- Honeydew
- Kiwi
- Mangos
- Oranges
- Peaches
- Prunes

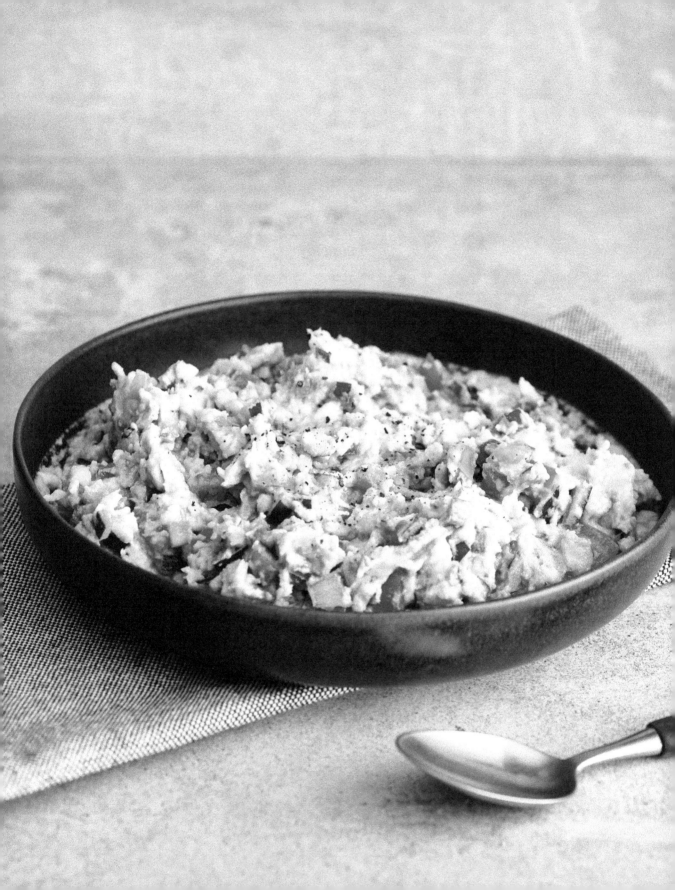

staples, sauces & dressings

Opposite: Guacamole, page 18

RED PEPPER DRY RUB

— MAKES ABOUT ¼ CUP —

I love to use this rub liberally on meat; it's so simple and adds great flavor. I created the recipe by adapting one my dad used to make when I was a little girl (his included brown sugar). I use this rub on steaks, pork chops, roasts, or chicken. You can also mix it with olive oil for more of a marinade. Let the meat marinate (either dry or with oil) in the refrigerator for 6 to 8 hours before cooking.

PREP TIME: 10 MINUTES

– ONE POT

– NO COOK

– 30 MINUTES

2 teaspoons red pepper flakes

2 teaspoons salt

1½ teaspoons granulated garlic

1½ teaspoons onion powder

1½ teaspoons freshly ground black pepper

1 teaspoon dry mustard

1 teaspoon ground cumin

½ teaspoon cloves

½ teaspoon dried sage

In a small bowl or jar, combine the red pepper flakes, salt, granulated garlic, onion powder, pepper, dry mustard, cumin, cloves, and sage. Use immediately or store in an airtight container.

SIMPLIFY IT! Make a large batch of this dry rub and keep it in your pantry. It will last for months and can be used on all sorts of proteins.

PER SERVING (1 TEASPOON)
Macronutrients: Fat 0%; Protein 0%; Carbs 100%
Calories: 6; Total Fat: 0g; Protein: 0g; Total Carbs: 1g; Fiber: 0g; Net Carbs: 1g

EVERYTHING MARINADE

— MAKES ABOUT ½ CUP —

I use this marinade on everything, hence the name. It's especially great on chicken and seafood. Marinades are incredibly versatile—you can make them with just about anything you like. Simply pick your favorite spices and add a little oil. It boosts healthy fats in your favorite dish and adds variety to your usual rotation.

PREP TIME: 10 MINUTES

– ONE POT

– NO COOK

– 30 MINUTES

– 5 INGREDIENTS

6 tablespoons olive oil

3 tablespoons white vinegar

1 teaspoon red pepper flakes

1 teaspoon whole-grain mustard

1 teaspoon salt

1 teaspoon freshly ground black pepper

1 teaspoon minced garlic

In a small bowl or large zip-top bag, mix the oil, vinegar, red pepper flakes, mustard, salt, pepper, and garlic. Use immediately or store in an airtight container for up to 2 weeks.

VARIATION TIP: Use this as a dressing on any type of salad, or use it as a marinade by tossing it with a pound of meat and refrigerating for at least an hour before cooking.

PER SERVING (1 TABLESPOON)
Macronutrients: Fat 100%; Protein 0%; Carbs 0%
Calories: 93; Total Fat: 11g; Protein: 0g; Total Carbs: 0g; Fiber: 0g; Net Carbs: 0g

LEMON-GARLIC DRESSING

— MAKES ABOUT ¾ CUP —

A tangy lemon vinaigrette is a great thing to have in the fridge. You can use it to dress a crisp green salad, as a dip for raw or steamed vegetables, or even as a marinade for meat. This is a simple recipe that can be easily dressed up by adding fresh herbs (try oregano, basil, or rosemary), mustard, or spices like ground cumin or paprika. You can also make it with lime instead of lemon.

PREP TIME: 10 MINUTES

- ONE POT
- NO COOK
- 30 MINUTES
- 5 INGREDIENTS

Zest and juice of 1 large lemon

6 garlic cloves, minced

1 teaspoon salt

1 teaspoon freshly ground black pepper

½ teaspoon Swerve granular (or other granulated alternative sweetener)

¾ cup olive oil

1 In a small bowl, whisk together the lemon zest and juice, garlic, salt, pepper, and sweetener.

2 While whisking, add the olive oil in a thin stream and whisk until the mixture emulsifies. Use immediately or store in an airtight container in the refrigerator for up to 2 weeks.

PER SERVING (2 TABLESPOONS)

Macronutrients: Fat 100%; Protein 0%; Carbs 0%
Calories: 223; Total Fat: 25g; Protein: 0g; Total Carbs: 2g; Fiber: 0g; Net Carbs: 2g

PICO DE GALLO

Pico de gallo might be my favorite food. It's colorful, full of spice, and so easy to make! I love serving it on top of eggs or with tacos (in a lettuce-wrap shell, of course). I could just about eat it straight from the bowl.

PREP TIME: 15 MINUTES

- ONE POT
- NO COOK
- 30 MINUTES
- 5 INGREDIENTS

1 large jalapeño pepper, diced

½ red onion, diced

10 cherry tomatoes, diced

8 garlic cloves, minced

3 tablespoons avocado oil

1½ teaspoons salt

½ teaspoon freshly ground black pepper

1 In a small bowl, combine the jalapeño, onion, tomatoes, and garlic.

2 Add the avocado oil, salt, and black pepper, and mix to combine. Serve immediately or store in an airtight container in the refrigerator for up to 5 days.

INGREDIENT TIP: If you prefer a milder salsa, omit the jalapeño or only use half a pepper.

PER SERVING (¼ CUP)
Macronutrients: Fat 74%; Protein 6%; Carbs 20%
Calories: 61; Total Fat: 5g; Protein: 1g; Total Carbs: 3g; Fiber: 1g; Net Carbs: 2g

GUACAMOLE

— MAKES 2½ CUPS —

I love splitting this guacamole recipe down the middle and making half super spicy and the other half mild (just omit the jalapeño from the mild side). It's great with fresh vegetables for dipping; my favorites are cucumbers, celery, tomatoes, and thinly sliced radish chips. Create a festive appetizer platter by layering guacamole on chunks of celery and topping each one with a spoonful of Pico de Gallo (page 17).

PREP TIME: 20 MINUTES

- ONE POT
- NO COOK
- 30 MINUTES
- 5 INGREDIENTS

3 avocados, halved, pitted, and peeled

½ red onion, diced

1 small tomato, diced

1 jalapeño pepper, diced (optional)

1 teaspoon garlic salt

½ teaspoon freshly ground black pepper

1 In a small bowl, mash the avocados with a fork until desired consistency is achieved. (I prefer my guacamole chunky.)

2 Add the onion, tomato, and jalapeño (if using), and stir to combine.

3 Add the garlic salt and black pepper. Stir and serve immediately.

SIMPLIFY IT! Already have your Pico de Gallo (page 17) made? Add some to the mashed avocados and voilà: ready-made guacamole.

PER SERVING (½ CUP)
Macronutrients: Fat 72%; Protein 6%; Carbs 22%
Calories: 200; Total Fat: 16g; Protein: 3g;
Total Carbs: 11g; Fiber: 8g; Net Carbs: 3g;
Erythritol 0.5g

EASIEST TARTAR SAUCE

— MAKES ABOUT 1 CUP —

Creamy tartar sauce studded with pickles is the perfect partner for certain seafood dishes, especially fried or grilled fish or seafood, but commercial brands (and many restaurant versions) often contain sugar. This DIY tartar sauce is totally keto friendly. Serve it alongside a meal of Salmon Patties (page 90), Country Club Crab Cakes (page 91), or "Fried" Oysters in the Oven (page 97).

PREP TIME: 5 MINUTES

- ONE POT
- NO COOK
- 30 MINUTES
- 5 INGREDIENTS

1 cup sugar-free mayonnaise (like Primal Kitchen)

3 tablespoons chopped dill pickles

1 teaspoon yellow mustard

1 teaspoon Swerve granular (or other granulated alternative sweetener)

1 In a small bowl or jar, whisk or shake together the mayonnaise, pickles, mustard, and sweetener.

2 Use immediately or store in an airtight container in the refrigerator for up to 1 week.

VARIATION TIP: This simple sauce uses just a few ingredients to deliver a ton of flavor, but you can make it even more delicious by adding minced fresh dill, chopped capers, or minced chives or shallots.

PER SERVING (2 TABLESPOONS)
Macronutrients: Fat 98%; Protein 0%; Carbs 2%
Calories: 211; Total Fat: 23g; Protein: 0g; Total Carbs: 1g; Fiber: 0g; Net Carbs: 1g

PICKLED CUCUMBERS AND ONIONS

— SERVES 6 —

My Aunt Mop used to make this, and I'll always remember her asking, "Want some cukes and onions, Jess?" I love to serve this alongside a bunless burger at lunchtime. It's also great as a salad topper or mixed with tuna or salmon and sugar-free mayonnaise for a quick fish salad.

PREP TIME: 10 MINUTES

– ONE POT

– NO COOK

– 30 MINUTES

– 5 INGREDIENTS

5 or 6 baby cucumbers, diced

1 large white onion, diced

1 cup white vinegar

2 teaspoons chopped fresh dill

1½ teaspoons salt

1 teaspoon freshly ground black pepper

1 teaspoon olive oil

In a mason jar or other airtight container, combine the cucumbers, onion, vinegar, dill, salt, pepper, and olive oil. Serve immediately, or cover and store in the refrigerator for up to 2 weeks.

PER SERVING

Macronutrients: Fat 22%; Protein 10%; Carbs 68%
Calories: 62; Total Fat: 2g; Protein: 2g; Total Carbs: 10g; Fiber: 2g; Net Carbs: 8g

MACADAMIA NUT BUTTER

— MAKES ABOUT 1 CUP —

Once, we ran out of my husband's favorite almond butter, but we happened
to have salted macadamia nuts in the pantry. I whipped up this smooth,
salty, complex nut butter, and ever since, Brad asks me to make it about
once a week. You can double or even triple the size of the batch if you
find that it disappears as quickly in your house as it does in mine.

PREP TIME: 10 MINUTES

– ONE POT
– NO COOK
– 30 MINUTES
– 5 INGREDIENTS

**1 (8-ounce) bag salted
macadamia nuts**

**1 teaspoon Swerve granular (or other
granulated alternative sweetener)**

1 In a blender or food processor, combine the
macadamia nuts and sweetener, and pulse until
the desired consistency is achieved.

2 Store in an airtight container in the refrigerator for up to 2 weeks.

INGREDIENT TIP: Use unsalted macadamia
nuts if you're watching your sodium—this recipe
tastes great either way.

PER SERVING (1 TABLESPOON)
Macronutrients: Fat 89%; Protein 4%; Carbs 7%
Calories: 111; Total Fat: 11g; Protein: 1g; Total
Carbs: 2g; Fiber: 1g; Net Carbs: 1g; Erythritol 0.5g

CREAM CHEESE ICING

— MAKES ABOUT 1½ CUPS —

This is going to be your new go-to icing; try to resist eating it by the spoonful. Use it as a dip for strawberries, blackberries, or blueberries, or get really decadent and serve it with my Best Brownies (page 144).

PREP TIME: 10 MINUTES

– ONE POT

– NO COOK

– 30 MINUTES

– 5 INGREDIENTS

1 (8-ounce) container dairy-free cream cheese (such as Kite Hill), at room temperature

¼ cup Swerve confectioners' (or other powdered alternative sweetener)

1 teaspoon vanilla extract

In a small bowl, blend together the cream cheese, sweetener, and vanilla. Use immediately or refrigerate to stiffen. Store covered in the refrigerator for up to 1 week.

PER SERVING (2 TABLESPOONS)

Macronutrients: Fat 76%; Protein 6%; Carbs 18%
Calories: 68; Total Fat: 4g; Protein: 1g; Total Carbs: 3g; Fiber: 0g; Net Carbs: 3g; Erythritol 4g

CHOCOLATE SAUCE

— MAKES ABOUT 1 CUP —

I love this chocolate sauce because it's both foolproof and versatile. Dip strawberries in it while it's still hot and then freeze on a baking sheet, drizzle it over coconut milk ice cream, or create a blissful keto candy bar: Simply add nuts, bacon bits, and pink Himalayan salt, and freeze on a rimmed baking sheet.

PREP TIME: 10 MINUTES

COOK TIME: 15 MINUTES

– ONE POT

– 30 MINUTES

– 5 INGREDIENTS

1 cup cacao butter

1 heaping tablespoon raw cacao powder (see tip)

2 tablespoons Swerve confectioners' (or other powdered alternative sweetener)

1 In a small saucepan, melt the cacao butter over medium-low heat.

2 While stirring continuously, add the cacao powder and sweetener. Cook, stirring, until the sweetener is dissolved, about 15 minutes.

3 Serve hot for dipping, store in an airtight container in the refrigerator for up to 2 weeks, or freeze for up to 3 months.

INGREDIENT TIP: Ever wondered what the difference is between "cocoa" and "cacao" products? Both are made from the same beans, but *cocoa* products generally come from beans that have been roasted at high temperatures, while *cacao* products are considered "raw" in that they are never heated above 115ºF during the production process.

PER SERVING (1 TABLESPOON)

Macronutrients: Fat 97%; Protein 2%; Carbs 1%
Calories: 133; Total Fat: 14g; Protein: 1g; Total
Carbs: 0.5g; Fiber: 0g; Net Carbs: 0.5g

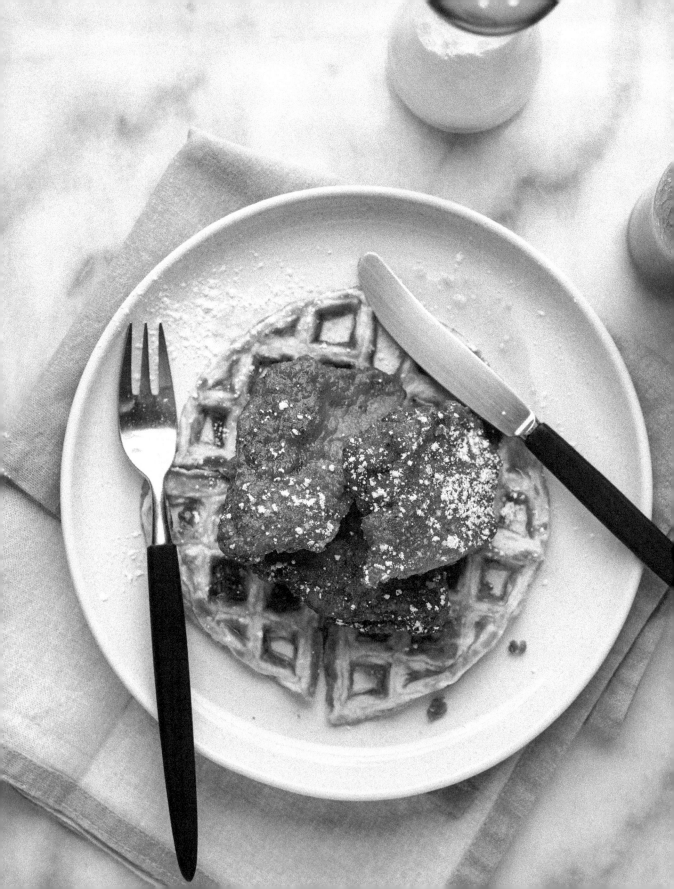

breakfast & brunch

Opposite: Hot Chicken and Waffles, page 41

KETO FAUX CAPPUCCINO

— SERVES 1 —

I love waking up to a frothy, creamy cup of coffee. Using a combination of nut milk, edible collagen, and MCT (medium-chain triglycerides) oil powder, I can have the morning "cappuccino" I love without the dairy. I use an electric frother, which heats and froths the nut milk, collagen, and MCT oil powder at the same time. You can also use a handheld frothing wand (around $10 will get you a good one); simply heat the mixture in the microwave for about 20 seconds first.

PREP TIME: 10 MINUTES

– ONE POT

– NO COOK

– 30 MINUTES

– 5 INGREDIENTS

¼ cup nut milk (I love Nutpods hazelnut)

1 scoop vanilla-flavored collagen (I recommend Primal Kitchen)

1 scoop MCT oil powder (I recommend Perfect Keto)

1 cup brewed coffee

1 Combine the nut milk, collagen, and MCT oil powder in an electric frother or a coffee cup. Froth until fluffy and thick. (If using a handheld frother, heat the mixture for about 20 seconds in the microwave beforehand.)

2 Combine the froth mixture with the coffee and enjoy immediately.

INGREDIENT TIP: If you're new to MCT oil powder, too much at once can cause stomach discomfort. I recommend starting with ¼ scoop and gradually increasing the amount over time.

PER SERVING

Macronutrients: Fat 58%; Protein 28%; Carbs 14%
Calories: 183; Total Fat: 11g; Protein: 13g; Total Carbs: 6g; Fiber: 2g; Net Carbs: 4g

CAULIFLOWER OATMEAL WITH BLUEBERRIES

— SERVES 2 —

Oatmeal! Oh, how I miss it. But my trusty friend cauliflower has served me well as a replacement for everything carb-y—including oatmeal. Cauliflower has a unique ability to take on any flavor (and even texture), and with this recipe, you'd never know you were eating a bowl of maple-and-coconut cruciferous vegetables. Believe it or not, I've even come to prefer this version over the original. Add a spoonful of raw cacao butter on top while everything is still hot. It will melt into the mixture and add richness.

PREP TIME: 5 MINUTES

COOK TIME: 15 MINUTES

– ONE POT

– 30 MINUTES

1 (12-ounce) bag riced cauliflower

1 (14-ounce) can coconut milk

2 tablespoons walnut oil

2 tablespoons peanut butter powder

2 tablespoons sugar-free maple syrup (such as ChocZero)

10 blueberries

1 In a medium saucepan, combine the cauliflower and coconut milk and bring to a boil over medium-high heat.

2 Reduce the heat to medium-low and stir in the walnut oil, peanut butter powder, and syrup. Cook, stirring occasionally, for 10 minutes.

3 Serve immediately, topped with the blueberries.

INGREDIENT TIP: ChocZero's line of Honest Syrups use alternative sweeteners; their maple syrup is sweetened with monk fruit.

PER SERVING

Macronutrients: Fat 79%; Protein 5%; Carbs 16%
Calories: 684; Total Fat: 60g; Protein: 9g; Total Carbs: 27g; Fiber: 10g; Net Carbs: 17g

CHIA SEED BREAKFAST BOWL

— SERVES 2 —

Chia seeds are a nutrient-dense food loaded with healthy omega-3 fatty acids, protein, fiber, antioxidants, and calcium. Their mild, nutty flavor makes them easy to add to a variety of foods. They can also absorb about 10 times their volume in liquid, so when you soak them in water, they become a gel that serves as a great thickening agent when you're avoiding more traditional thickeners like flour and dairy products. This breakfast bowl with fresh berries is one of my favorite ways to enjoy chia seeds—I eat it a few mornings every week.

PREP TIME: 5 MINUTES (PLUS 3 HOURS TO CHILL)

– ONE POT

– NO COOK

– 5 INGREDIENTS

1¼ cups canned coconut milk

¼ cup chia seeds

½ cup fresh berries, such as strawberries and blueberries

1 In an airtight container, mix together the coconut milk and chia seeds. Chill in the refrigerator for at least 3 hours or overnight.

2 Just before serving, add the berries.

VARIATION TIP: The berries make this pretty sweet, but if you like your breakfast even sweeter, add a bit of low-carb syrup or alternative sweetener like Swerve.

PER SERVING

Macronutrients: Fat 78%; Protein 6%; Carbs 16%
Calories: 389; Total Fat: 36g; Protein: 6g; Total Carbs: 16g; Fiber: 8g; Net Carbs: 8g

YOGURT BOWL WITH BERRIES

— SERVES 1 —

When I discovered dairy-free yogurt, I felt like I had won the lottery. Rich, creamy yogurt studded with sweet fresh berries makes such a satisfying breakfast on mornings when I don't feel like cooking anything. The walnut oil and coconut flakes add complexity and texture. Skip the berries if you want to keep your carbs down.

PREP TIME: 10 MINUTES

– ONE POT
– NO COOK
– 30 MINUTES

½ cup dairy-free plain yogurt (such as Kite Hill)

10 blueberries

4 strawberries, diced

1 tablespoon unsweetened fresh coconut flakes

1 teaspoon vanilla extract

1 teaspoon walnut oil

1 teaspoon Swerve granular (or other granulated alternative sweetener)

In a small bowl, mix together the yogurt, blueberries, strawberries, coconut flakes, vanilla extract, walnut oil, and sweetener. Serve immediately.

PER SERVING

Macronutrients: Fat 49%; Protein 10%; Carbs 41%

Calories: 140; Total Fat: 7g; Protein: 4g;

Total Carbs: 18g; Fiber: 0g; Net Carbs: 18g;

Erythritol 4g

WAFFLES

— MAKES 6 WAFFLES —

Waffles are such a treat on a weekend morning—or, really, any morning. Believe it or not, dairy-free, keto-friendly waffles are delicious and every bit as easy to make as the high-carb, dairy-full version. The key to cooking them just right is to barely cover the waffle iron with the batter (use about ¼ cup of batter per waffle). Ideally, you want a layer so thin you can still see the squares of the waffle iron through it.

PREP TIME: 10 MINUTES

COOK TIME: 20 MINUTES

− 30 MINUTES

− 5 INGREDIENTS

1 (8-ounce) container of dairy-free cream cheese (such as Kite Hill)

7 large eggs

1½ tablespoons cinnamon

4 teaspoons Swerve granular (or other granulated alternative sweetener)

2 tablespoons olive oil, divided

Sugar-free maple-flavored syrup (I love ChocZero), for serving

1 In a large microwave-safe bowl, heat the cream cheese in the microwave for 45 seconds. Use a wire whisk to whip until fluffy.

2 Add the eggs and continue to whip until the mixture is well combined and thick. Stir in the cinnamon, sweetener, and 1 tablespoon of oil.

3 Liberally grease the waffle iron with the remaining 1 tablespoon of oil and pour the batter in the iron ¼ cup at a time. Cook according to the waffle iron manufacturer's instructions.

4 Serve hot, topped with syrup.

VARIATION TIP: I also like these sprinkled with a little powdered sweetener and drizzled with walnut oil.

PER SERVING (1 WAFFLE)

Macronutrients: Fat 79%; Protein 16%; Carbs 5%

Calories: 227; Total Fat: 19g; Protein: 9g; Total Carbs: 3g; Fiber: 0g; Net Carbs: 3g; Erythritol 2g

PERFECT BACON

— SERVES 4 —

Can you ever go wrong with perfectly cooked bacon? The answer is no. Oven baking will be your favorite way to cook bacon from here on out. Thanks to parchment paper, cleanup is easy, too. I recommend cooking up Homestyle Fried Eggs (page 32) just before the bacon is ready to come out of the oven.

PREP TIME: 5 MINUTES

COOK TIME: 22 MINUTES

– ONE POT

– 30 MINUTES

– 5 INGREDIENTS

1 (12-ounce) package bacon (8 to 12 strips)

1 Preheat the oven to 400°F.

2 Line a large baking sheet with two pieces of parchment paper.

3 Arrange the bacon strips in a single layer on the prepared sheet.

4 Cook in the preheated oven for 22 minutes.

5 Let cool slightly before serving.

VARIATION TIP: For a sweet-savory surprise, spread a little Macadamia Nut Butter (page 21) on top of each bacon strip after it has cooled.

PER SERVING

Macronutrients: Fat 72%; Protein 28%; Carbs 0%
Calories: 100; Total Fat: 8g; Protein: 7g; Total Carbs: 0g; Fiber: 0g; Net Carbs: 0g

HOMESTYLE FRIED EGGS

— MAKES 2 EGGS —

I don't mean to brag, but I can fry an egg. This no-fail method will give you the most picture-perfect fried eggs, too. It's all about the oil, which prevents them from sticking to the pan so that they fry perfectly. Just be forewarned, once word gets out about these, people might start randomly showing up at your house for breakfast.

PREP TIME: 2 MINUTES

COOK TIME: 5 MINUTES

- ONE POT
- 30 MINUTES
- 5 INGREDIENTS

3 tablespoons olive oil or avocado oil

2 large eggs

1 teaspoon salt

½ teaspoon freshly ground black pepper

1 In a small skillet over high heat, heat the oil, tilting the pan to coat.

2 Crack the eggs into the hot oil. Season with the salt and pepper.

3 Remove from the heat, and let the eggs continue to cook for about 3 minutes, until the whites are set and the edges are browned and crisp. Serve hot.

PER SERVING (2 EGGS)
Macronutrients: Fat 86%; Protein 13%; Carbs 1%
Calories: 382; Total Fat: 37g; Protein: 13g; Total Carbs: 1g; Fiber: 0g; Net Carbs: 1g

CRUSTLESS QUICHE WITH HAM, MUSHROOMS, AND ONION

— SERVES 8 —

What is it about a quiche that screams fancy? I think it's the word *quiche* alone. Whenever I make one, I feel like it's an open invitation to have friends over, pour some coffee, and gather around the table with thick wedges of this vegetable-laden dish. I like to serve it with a side of Perfect Bacon (page 31).

PREP TIME: 20 MINUTES

COOK TIME: 1 HOUR 10 MINUTES

2 tablespoons olive oil, plus more for greasing the pie plate

10 large eggs

2 cups diced ham

1 cup mushrooms

1 white onion, diced

½ cup canned coconut milk

1 tablespoon garlic powder

1 teaspoon salt

½ teaspoon freshly ground black pepper

2 tablespoons minced fresh chives

1 Preheat the oven to 400°F.

2 Grease a 9-inch glass pie plate.

3 In a large mixing bowl, stir together the eggs, ham, mushrooms, onion, coconut milk, olive oil, garlic powder, salt, and pepper. Pour the mixture into the greased pie plate.

4 Bake for 1 hour 10 minutes, until the center is set and the top is golden brown.

5 Serve immediately, garnished with the chives, or wrap and store in the refrigerator for up to 1 week.

PER SERVING

Macronutrients: Fat 65%; Protein 25%; Carbs 10%

Calories: 220; Total Fat: 16g; Protein: 14g; Total Carbs: 5g; Fiber: 2g; Net Carbs: 3g

SUN-DRIED TOMATO AND HAM OMELET

— SERVES 2 —

I love to make a huge, veggie-stuffed omelet to split with Brad. There's something about an omelet that looks and feels just right: You know instantly that it will be a satisfying and energizing meal because it's loaded with protein and good fat content. Plus it's easy and customizable.

PREP TIME: 5 MINUTES

COOK TIME: 15 MINUTES

– 30 MINUTES

– 5 INGREDIENTS

6 large eggs

½ cup canned coconut milk

1 teaspoon salt

1 teaspoon freshly ground
black pepper

¼ cup coconut oil

½ cup fresh spinach

¾ cup diced ham

2 tablespoons sun-dried tomatoes

1 In a small bowl, whisk together the eggs, milk, salt, and pepper.

2 Heat the oil in a medium skillet over medium heat. Add the egg mixture and reduce the heat to medium-low.

3 Once the egg mixture begins to bubble on the sides, add the spinach, ham, and sun-dried tomatoes, and cook for 3 minutes.

4 Using a spatula, fold over the eggs once to make a half-moon shape.

5 Flip carefully and continue cooking for 3 to 5 additional minutes.

6 Transfer to a plate and serve.

VARIATION TIP: You can add all sorts of things to your omelet. Try chopped fresh herbs, diced bell peppers, chopped tomatoes, onion, shallot, or mushrooms.

PER SERVING

Macronutrients: Fat 76%; Protein 21%; Carbs 3%
Calories: 646; Total Fat: 54g; Protein: 30g; Total
Carbs: 5g; Fiber: 3g; Net Carbs: 2g

RUSTIC EGG BITES

— MAKES 12 —

When I happen to have a refrigerator full of these miniature two-bite breakfast snacks, I sometimes eat them for breakfast, lunch, and dinner. I add sausage because it makes them especially filling and hearty. They're great warm from the oven, reheated, or even straight out of the refrigerator.

PREP TIME: 20 MINUTES

COOK TIME: 22 MINUTES

– 5 INGREDIENTS

1 tablespoon avocado oil, plus more for greasing the muffin tin

1 pound ground sausage

12 large eggs

⅔ cup canned coconut milk

2 tablespoons minced garlic

1 tablespoon salsa

1 teaspoon salt

½ teaspoon freshly ground black pepper

1 Preheat the oven to 400°F. Grease a 12-cup muffin tin with oil.

2 In a large skillet over medium-high heat, cook the sausage, stirring and breaking up the meat with a spatula, until browned, about 5 minutes. Remove from the heat and let cool for a few minutes.

3 Crack the eggs into a medium mixing bowl and add the coconut milk, garlic, salsa, avocado oil, salt, and pepper. Whisk to combine.

4 Stir the cooked sausage into the egg mixture, then pour the mixture evenly into the prepared muffin tin. Bake in the preheated oven for 25 minutes.

5 Serve warm or store in an airtight container in the refrigerator for up to 1 week.

SUBSTITUTION TIP: You can replace the sausage with cooked bacon and add any vegetables you like, such as diced bell pepper or jalapeño, or halved cherry tomatoes.

PER SERVING (1 EGG)

Macronutrients: Fat 70%; Protein 25%; Carbs 5%

Calories: 243; Total Fat: 19g; Protein: 15g; Total Carbs: 3g; Fiber: 0g; Net Carbs: 3g

MONTE CRISTO SANDWICHES

— MAKES 6 SANDWICHES —

One day not long ago, Brad said, "You should make Monte Cristo sandwiches with your waffle recipe!" Truth be told, I had never even heard of a Monte Cristo sandwich. After a little research, I couldn't believe I had missed out on this goodness all my life. A classic Monte Cristo is a ham-and-cheese sandwich, dipped in egg and fried. And yes, I did figure out how to make a version that is both dairy-free and keto.

PREP TIME: 10 MINUTES

COOK TIME: 10 MINUTES

– 30 MINUTES

– 5 INGREDIENTS

6 large eggs

1 teaspoon salt

1 teaspoon freshly ground black pepper

2 tablespoons olive oil

1 recipe Waffles (page 30)

1 recipe Perfect Bacon (page 31)

¼ cup low-carb syrup (like ChocZero)

6 tablespoons Swerve confectioners' (or other powdered alternative sweetener)

1 In a small bowl, whisk together the eggs, salt, and pepper.

2 In a small skillet, heat the oil over medium heat. Add the egg mixture and cook, stirring continuously, until thoroughly cooked, about 6 minutes.

3 Top half of each waffle with some of the scrambled egg and 2 or 3 pieces of bacon. Fold the waffle over to make a sandwich and drizzle the syrup over the top. Sprinkle with the powdered sweetener and serve immediately.

PER SERVING (1 SANDWICH)

Macronutrients: Fat 74%; Protein 21%; Carbs 5%

Calories: 545; Total Fat: 45g; Protein: 29g;

Total Carbs: 13g; Fiber: 2g; Net Carbs: 11g;

Erythritol 12g

RADISH HASH BROWNS WITH ONION AND GREEN PEPPER

— SERVES 3 —

On keto, radishes are the new potatoes. It's amazing what you can do to transform the sharp tang of a red radish into the creamy smoothness of a baked potato dish. Southern staple Waffle House is known for its smothered, covered hash browns, and that's the dish that inspired me here. My version is smothered and covered, but good for you! It makes a nice, hearty breakfast topped with sugar-free ketchup (I like Primal Kitchen).

PREP TIME: 5 MINUTES

COOK TIME: 25 MINUTES

– ONE POT

– 30 MINUTES

– 5 INGREDIENTS

5 tablespoons olive oil

12 radishes, thinly sliced

1 onion, diced

1 green bell pepper, seeded and diced

6 garlic cloves, minced

1 teaspoon cayenne

1 teaspoon salt

½ teaspoon freshly ground black pepper

1 In a skillet over medium heat, heat the oil. Add the radishes, onion, bell pepper, and garlic. Cook, stirring frequently, until the vegetables are tender, about 5 minutes.

2 Add the cayenne, salt, and pepper. Continue to cook, stirring occasionally, for about 20 minutes, or until the vegetables are browned and crisp around the edges.

SUBSTITUTION TIP: If you don't have radishes, substitute cauliflower or turnips.

PER SERVING

Macronutrients: Fat 86%; Protein 1%; Carbs 13%

Calories: 252; Total Fat: 24g; Protein: 1g; Total Carbs: 8g; Fiber: 2g; Net Carbs: 6g

SAUSAGE BREAKFAST HASH

— SERVES 6 —

Sausage hash makes a fantastic and filling breakfast, and it's a nice break from eggs—though it's also great with a couple of poached or fried eggs on top. It's got all the ingredients of a one-pan breakfast, and it's also ideal for those late nights after a hectic day, when all you can manage is breakfast for dinner.

PREP TIME: 15 MINUTES

COOK TIME: 35 MINUTES

– ONE POT

6 tablespoons olive oil

1 pound kielbasa, cut into ½-inch pieces

1 green bell pepper, seeded and chopped

1 red bell pepper, seeded and chopped

1 red onion, diced

1 jalapeño pepper, diced

3 garlic cloves, minced

1 teaspoon salt

½ teaspoon freshly ground black pepper

1 (14-ounce) can stewed tomatoes

1 In a large skillet, heat the oil over medium heat. Add the kielbasa and cook, stirring, until browned, about 5 minutes.

2 Add the green pepper, red pepper, onion, jalapeño, garlic, salt, and black pepper. Cook, stirring occasionally, for 10 to 12 minutes, until the vegetables are softened and browned.

3 Reduce the heat to medium-low, stir in the tomatoes, cover, and let simmer for 15 minutes. Serve hot.

SUBSTITUTION TIP: You can substitute another type of sausage for the kielbasa, as long as it doesn't have sugar or other non-keto fillers in it. I like andouille or linguica.

PER SERVING

Macronutrients: Fat 74%; Protein 13%; Carbs 13%
Calories: 331; Total Fat: 27g; Protein: 11g; Total Carbs: 11g; Fiber: 2g; Net Carbs: 9g

DAD'S SAUSAGE GRAVY

— SERVES 8 —

One of my favorite memories of my dad is watching him make his special sausage gravy. I remember him standing at the stove over the cast iron skillet, wooden spoon in hand, stirring diligently. Mom would already have the biscuits in the oven. It's something I'll never have a photograph of, but I don't need one—the mental picture is preserved perfectly. This recipe uses alternative flours (almond and amaranth) to thicken the gravy without adding the carbs of all-purpose white flour. Amaranth flour is gluten-free and tastes similar to whole-wheat or rice flour—you can find it at specialty and gourmet grocery stores, as well as online. Serve this over biscuits and eggs, or with any other dish that calls for a rich, creamy gravy.

PREP TIME: 10 MINUTES

COOK TIME: 20 MINUTES

– ONE POT

– 30 MINUTES

2 tablespoons olive oil

1 pound pork sausage

½ white onion, diced

1 tablespoon minced garlic

1 (14-ounce) can coconut milk

¼ cup almond flour

1 teaspoon amaranth flour

1 teaspoon salt

½ teaspoon freshly ground pepper

1 In a cast iron skillet, heat the oil over medium-high heat. Add the sausage and cook, stirring and breaking up the meat with a spatula, until it begins to brown, about 2 minutes.

2 Add the onion and garlic, and continue to cook, stirring frequently, until the sausage is browned and the onion is soft, about 5 minutes.

3 Reduce the heat to medium and clear a space in the center of the meat mixture. Pour the coconut milk into the space. Then, stirring the milk constantly, add the almond and amaranth flours.

4 Cook, stirring, until the milk and flours are well combined, about 5 minutes.

5 Now stir the milk mixture and the meat together to mix well, and cook for another 3 to 5 minutes, or until thickened. Don't be alarmed if the texture is thinner than what you might be used to; it will still taste like an old-school, rich, creamy gravy.

6 Season with the salt and pepper, and serve hot.

CONTINUED →

DAD'S SAUSAGE GRAVY

continued

INGREDIENT TIP: When buying sausage, be sure to read the ingredients. Many sausage mixtures include cheese, sugar, or fillers that are not keto friendly. If you can't find sausage without fillers, substitute with your favorite ground meat, adding ½ teaspoon cayenne pepper, ½ teaspoon dried sage, ¼ teaspoon dried cumin, and an additional ½ teaspoon each of salt and freshly ground pepper. You won't even know the difference!

PER SERVING

Macronutrients: Fat 83%; Protein 12%; Carbs 5%
Calories: 335; Total Fat: 31g; Protein: 10g; Total Carbs: 4g; Fiber: 1g; Net Carbs: 3g

VARIATION TIP: Add ½ teaspoon cayenne pepper and/or an additional ½ teaspoon freshly ground black pepper to make it extra spicy; this is my favorite way to enjoy Dad's gravy.

HOT CHICKEN
AND WAFFLES

— SERVES 6 —

Nashville is famous for its hot chicken, and clever locals have paired the dish with waffles for as long as I can remember. As a Nashville resident, I'm proud to have taken the dish one step further with this keto-friendly alternative. Cook up this red-hot combo, and you'll be writing your next country tune in no time.

PREP TIME: 10 MINUTES

– ONE POT

– NO COOK

– 30 MINUTES

1 recipe Best Fried Chicken Ever (page 105)

¼ cup hot wing sauce (I like Frank's RedHot)

1 tablespoon cayenne

1 recipe Waffles (page 30)

6 tablespoons sugar-free maple-flavored syrup (such as ChocZero)

2 tablespoons Swerve confectioners' (or other powdered alternative sweetener)

1 In a bowl, toss the chicken in the hot sauce and cayenne.

2 Arrange the chicken on top of the waffles, drizzle the syrup over the top, sprinkle with powdered sweetener, and serve immediately.

PER SERVING

Macronutrients: Fat 76%; Protein 18%; Carbs 6%
Calories: 572; Total Fat: 48g; Protein: 26g;
Total Carbs: 22g; Fiber: 4g; Net Carbs: 18g;
Erythritol 6g

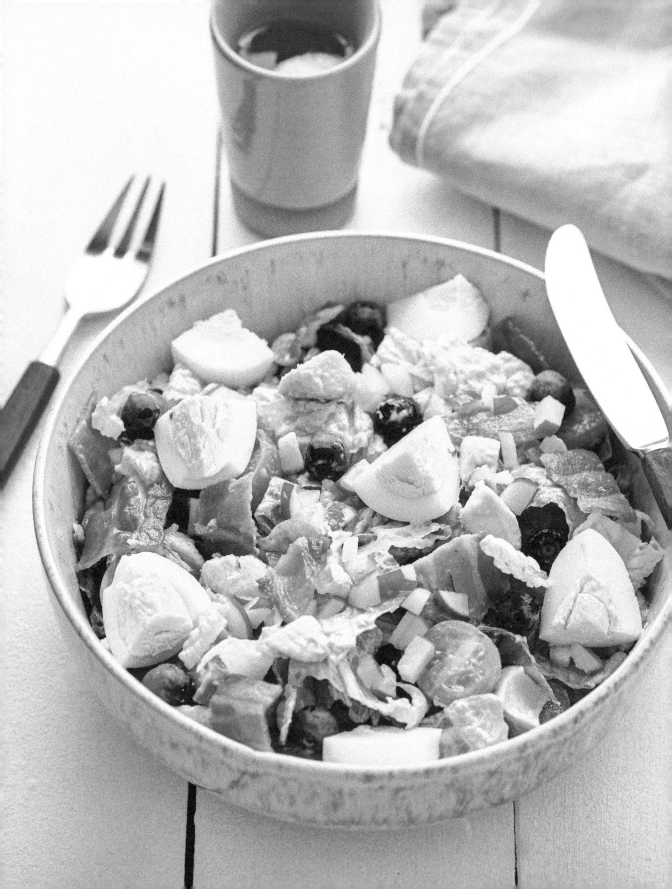

soups & salads

Opposite: Rainbow Chopped Salad, page 48

CAULIFLOWER AND BACON SOUP

— SERVES 8 —

In my pre–dairy-free keto days, I loved creamy potato soup with the delicate crunch of bacon bits. I even won a Girl Scouts cooking competition many moons ago with my potato-and-cheese version. So it was with high hopes and intense pressure that I tried to re-create the dish without cheese or cream, using cauliflower instead of potato. I don't know if my Brownie troop would approve, but I'm convinced this version is still a winner.

PREP TIME: 10 MINUTES

COOK TIME: 1 HOUR

1 head cauliflower, stemmed and cut into large pieces

2 (14-ounce) cans coconut milk

2 cups bone broth

6 tablespoons olive oil, divided

1 onion, diced

1 cup sliced mushrooms

6 garlic cloves, minced

1½ teaspoons salt

1½ teaspoons freshly ground black pepper

1½ teaspoons cayenne

1 batch Perfect Bacon, chopped or crumbled (page 31)

1 Fill a stockpot halfway with water and add the cauliflower. Bring to a boil and cook until the cauliflower is tender, about 20 minutes. Drain the cauliflower and then return it to the stockpot. Using a potato masher, mash the cauliflower until mostly smooth.

2 Put the pot over low heat, and add the coconut milk and broth.

3 In a separate skillet, heat 3 tablespoons of oil over medium heat. Add the onion, mushrooms, and garlic. Cook, stirring frequently, for 15 to 20 minutes, or until softened.

4 Add the onion mixture to the soup mixture and continue cooking over low heat for 5 to 7 more minutes.

5 Stir in the salt, pepper, cayenne, the remaining 3 tablespoons of oil, and the bacon. Cook for 20 minutes more.

6 Serve immediately or store the soup in an airtight container in the refrigerator for up to 1 week.

PER SERVING

Macronutrients: Fat 74%; Protein 18%; Carbs 8%
Calories: 414; Total Fat: 34g; Protein: 19g; Total Carbs: 8g; Fiber: 4g; Net Carbs: 4g

HEARTY VEGETABLE SOUP

— SERVES 8 —

Homemade soup may sound like a big undertaking, but with a slow cooker, it couldn't be easier. Just chop whatever vegetables you happen to have on hand and throw them in the pot with a few cups of broth. You can also make a giant batch and freeze it in individual servings; just take a portion out of the freezer whenever you want a comforting bowl of soup on demand.

PREP TIME: 30 MINUTES

COOK TIME: 8 HOURS

– ONE POT

8 cups vegetable broth

2 (14-ounce) cans diced tomatoes

1 (16-ounce) bag kale, chopped

1 bunch radishes (about 12), halved

1 onion, chopped

2 celery stalks, chopped

2 cups fresh or frozen green beans, cut into 2-inch pieces

1 cup whole mushrooms

4 garlic cloves, minced

¼ cup olive oil

1 In a slow cooker, combine the vegetable broth, tomatoes, kale, radishes, onion, celery, green beans, mushrooms, garlic, and olive oil.

2 Cover and cook on low for 8 hours. Serve hot.

VARIATION TIP: This is my favorite mix of veggies, but you can vary it based on what you have. Add broccoli, cauliflower, spinach, chard, turnips, or any other low-carb vegetables you like.

PER SERVING

Macronutrients: Fat 43%; Protein 21%; Carbs 36%

Calories: 168; Total Fat: 8g; Protein: 9g; Total Carbs: 15g; Fiber: 4g; Net Carbs: 11g

STUFFED-PEPPER SOUP

— SERVES 8 —

I make this soup whenever I'm craving stuffed peppers but can't be bothered to actually make them. It has all the flavors I love, and it's super easy to pull together. It freezes well, too, so I often make a double batch and store the leftovers in the freezer for easy heat-and-go meals. It will keep for up to 3 months in the freezer.

PREP TIME: 20 MINUTES

COOK TIME: 1 HOUR

− ONE POT

4 tablespoons olive oil, divided

1 pound ground beef

4 cups bone broth

1 (12-ounce) can tomato sauce

1 (12-ounce) bag riced cauliflower

1 (3.8-ounce) can diced black olives, drained

2 green bell peppers, diced

3 tablespoons minced garlic

1 In a large pot, heat 2 tablespoons of oil over medium-high heat. Add the beef and cook, stirring, until browned, about 5 minutes.

2 Add the broth, tomato sauce, cauliflower, olives, peppers, and garlic, and bring to a simmer.

3 Reduce the heat to low and let simmer for about 1 hour, or until the soup is thickened and the flavors have melded. Serve hot.

PER SERVING
Macronutrients: Fat 57%; Protein 32%; Carbs 11%
Calories: 286; Total Fat: 18g; Protein: 23g; Total Carbs: 8g; Fiber: 3g; Net Carbs: 5g

BROCCOLI SALAD

— SERVES 6 —

This is a great make-ahead salad. It stores well and tastes even better after it's been chilled in the refrigerator for a while. You can use chopped broccoli spears for this recipe, if you like, but I prefer the texture of the broccoli slaw, which you can buy already shredded to save on prep time.

PREP TIME: 10 MINUTES

– ONE POT

– NO COOK

– 30 MINUTES

1 (12-ounce) bag broccoli slaw (or 1 head broccoli, chopped or shredded)

1½ cups low-carb mayonnaise (like Primal Kitchen)

6 tablespoons salted sunflower seeds

½ cup chopped red onion

¼ cup white vinegar

4 strips Perfect Bacon (page 31), chopped

2 teaspoons Swerve granular (or other granulated alternative sweetener)

5 red grapes (optional)

1 In an airtight container, mix the broccoli slaw, mayonnaise, sunflower seeds, onion, vinegar, bacon, sweetener, and grapes (if using).

2 Cover and chill for at least 2 hours. Serve cold. Store in an airtight container in the refrigerator for up to 3 days.

VARIATION TIP: Swap in chopped salami for the bacon and add a pint of halved cherry tomatoes for an Italian-inspired version.

PER SERVING

Macronutrients: Fat 90%; Protein 5%; Carbs 5% Calories: 564; Total Fat: 56g; Protein: 7g; Total Carbs: 7g; Fiber: 2g; Net Carbs: 5g; Erythritol 1g

RAINBOW CHOPPED SALAD

— SERVES 1 —

I love the combination of sweet and savory in this chopped salad.
It's a beautiful example of a dish that delivers all kinds of nutrients
through green, red, pink, and even blue vegetables and fruits.

PREP TIME: 20 MINUTES

– ONE POT

– NO COOK

– 30 MINUTES

1 cup chopped romaine lettuce

1 avocado, halved, pitted, peeled,
and diced

2 No-Fail Hard-Boiled Eggs
(page 67), chopped

½ cup diced Perfect Bacon (page 31)

10 blueberries

4 small cherry tomatoes, halved

1 radish, chopped

1 breast of Slow-Cooker Buffalo
Chicken (page 102; optional)

¼ cup low-carb, dairy-free ranch
dressing (such as Tessemae's)

In a medium bowl, combine the lettuce,
avocado, eggs, bacon, blueberries, cherry
tomatoes, and radish. Add the chicken
(if using) and salad dressing, toss to combine,
and serve immediately.

VARIATION TIP: Adding the Slow-Cooker
Buffalo Chicken (page 102) makes this salad
a meal. The spiciness of the chicken perfectly
balances the sweetness of the blueberries and
tomatoes.

PER SERVING

Macronutrients: Fat 74%; Protein 16%; Carbs 10%
Calories: 864; Total Fat: 73g; Protein: 35g; Total
Carbs: 23g; Fiber: 13g; Net Carbs: 10g

WEDGE SALAD WITH RANCH DRESSING

— SERVES 4 —

I love a wedge salad more than just about anything. But sadly, the star of most wedge salads is dairy-heavy blue cheese dressing. That's where dairy-free ranch dressing comes in; I love the one made by Tessemae's. For a gourmet restaurant touch, chill the plates in the fridge for about 10 minutes ahead of time, so the salad remains super cold when served.

PREP TIME: 20 MINUTES

– ONE POT

– NO COOK

– 30 MINUTES

1 head iceberg lettuce, cut into 4 wedges

½ cup low-carb, dairy-free ranch dressing (such as Tessemae's)

6 tablespoons bacon bits

1 tomato, diced

4 radishes, diced

¼ cup chopped fresh chives

½ teaspoon freshly ground black pepper

Arrange the lettuce wedges on 4 serving plates. Top each wedge with 2 tablespoons of dressing. Add the bacon bits, tomato, radishes, chives, and pepper. Serve immediately.

PER SERVING

Macronutrients: Fat 76%; Protein 12%; Carbs 12%

Calories: 201; Total Fat: 17g; Protein: 6g; Total Carbs: 6g; Fiber: 1g; Net Carbs: 5g

COLD CAULIFLOWER "PASTA" SALAD

— SERVES 8 —

Cauliflower is a magic vegetable in the keto world. It's low in carbs but can be used as a substitute for lots of high-carb staples like rice, beans, potatoes, or even pasta. This simple, quick pasta-less "pasta" salad is my most requested recipe. The diced salami really makes it for me, but you could substitute diced cooked bacon or ham. When I have this in the fridge, I tend to eat it as is, straight out of the refrigerator, for lunch or dinner.

PREP TIME: 15 MINUTES (PLUS 2 HOURS 30 MINUTES TO CHILL)

– ONE POT

– 5 INGREDIENTS

2 (12-ounce) bags riced cauliflower

1 red bell pepper, seeded and diced

1 cup diced dried salami

1 cucumber, diced

¼ cup olive oil

2 tablespoons minced garlic

1 teaspoon salt

1 In the microwave, cook the cauliflower rice according to the package directions. Refrigerate for at least 30 minutes.

2 Add the bell pepper, salami, cucumber, olive oil, garlic, and salt. Mix well, then cover and refrigerate for at least 2 hours to chill.

3 Serve cold or store in an airtight container in the refrigerator for up to 1 week.

VARIATION TIP: Add other vegetables here if you like, such as diced tomatoes, diced green bell pepper, or even sliced peperoncini.

PER SERVING

Macronutrients: Fat 70%; Protein 16%; Carbs 14%
Calories: 208; Total Fat: 16g; Protein: 9g; Total Carbs: 7g; Fiber: 3g; Net Carbs: 4g

EGG SALAD WITH DILL

— SERVES 12 —

This egg salad is a perennial favorite, with just the right amount of kick from the paprika and fresh dill. It's a great salad to keep in the refrigerator for easy, anytime meal prep. It's got lots of healthy fats, and it can be used in many different ways. Try it on top of a green salad, wrapped in lettuce leaves, or as dip for raw vegetables. I like to add minced celery or a shake of curry powder for a change of pace.

PREP TIME: 30 MINUTES
(PLUS 2 HOURS TO CHILL)

– ONE POT

– NO COOK

– 5 INGREDIENTS

12 No-Fail Hard-Boiled Eggs (page 67), peeled and diced

1½ cups low-carb mayonnaise (such as Primal Kitchen)

1 teaspoon salt

1 teaspoon chopped fresh dill

1 teaspoon Swerve granular (or other granulated alternative sweetener)

½ teaspoon freshly ground black pepper

½ teaspoon paprika

1 In a medium bowl, combine the eggs, mayonnaise, salt, dill, sweetener, pepper, and paprika.

2 Cover and refrigerate for at least 2 hours. Serve cold. Store in an airtight container in the refrigerator for up to 1 week.

VARIATION TIP: Serve this with steamed vegetables and slices of salami or prosciutto for a snacky lunch or dinner. You can even use it as a topping for a burger!

PER SERVING

Macronutrients: Fat 90%; Protein 9%; Carbs 1%
Calories: 280; Total Fat: 28g; Protein: 6g; Total Carbs: 1g; Fiber: 0g; Net Carbs: 1g; Erythritol 0.5g

SIMPLE HAM SALAD

— SERVES 4 —

This salad is super simple—just ham, mayonnaise, and celery—but it really satisfies my appetite when I'm hungry and don't have time to cook. I sometimes make a triple batch on Sunday and eat it throughout the week. I like it scooped up with crunchy vegetables or wrapped in lettuce leaves. If you don't like mayonnaise, you can use dairy-free cream cheese instead.

PREP TIME: 10 MINUTES

- ONE POT
- NO COOK
- 30 MINUTES
- 5 INGREDIENTS

2 cups diced ham

¾ cup low-carb mayonnaise (such as Primal Kitchen)

2 celery stalks, diced

In a small bowl, combine the ham, mayonnaise, and celery, and stir to mix well. Serve immediately or store, covered, in the refrigerator for up to 1 week.

VARIATION TIP: This recipe is classic and plain, but it's easy to add some punch: Add a few tablespoons of chopped shallots or a couple of chopped dill pickles.

PER SERVING

Macronutrients: Fat 87%; Protein 10%; Carbs 3%
Calories: 434; Total Fat: 42g; Protein: 11g; Total Carbs: 3g; Fiber: 1g; Net Carbs: 2g

CHICKEN SALAD WITH GRAPES AND ALMONDS

— SERVES 8 —

This is the perfect chicken salad. I warn you—once you make it, your friends and family will never stop requesting it. Brad loves chicken salad, and this is another dish I like to have on hand for an easy meal. It's a great raid-the-pantry recipe, and you can use leftover chicken if you've got it. Serve the salad with a lettuce wedge, in lettuce cups, or paired with a serving of Egg Salad with Dill (page 51).

PREP TIME: 10 MINUTES

COOK TIME: 20 MINUTES

– 30 MINUTES

6 boneless, skinless chicken breasts

3 tablespoons olive oil

1½ cups sugar-free mayonnaise (such as Primal Kitchen)

½ cup diced celery

10 grapes, diced (optional)

¼ cup slivered almonds

3 tablespoons poppy seeds

1 tablespoon chopped fresh dill

1 tablespoon dry mustard

1 Place the chicken breasts in a stockpot and cover completely with water. Bring to a boil and cook until the chicken is cooked through. about 20 minutes. Drain.

2 Put the chicken in a blender or food processor with the olive oil. Pulse until the chicken is very finely chopped.

3 In a large bowl, combine the chicken with the mayonnaise, celery, grapes (if using), almonds, poppy seeds, dill, and mustard. Serve immediately or cover and refrigerate for up to 1 week.

SIMPLIFY IT! To skip step 1 and save time, you can use any leftover cooked chicken you have, or stop by the supermarket and pick up a rotisserie chicken.

PER SERVING

Macronutrients: Fat 81%; Protein 17%; Carbs 2%
Calories: 506; Total Fat: 46g; Protein: 21g; Total Carbs: 2g; Fiber: 1g; Net Carbs: 1g

SPICY SHRIMP SALAD

— SERVES 8 —

I like to keep the shrimp in this zesty seafood salad whole, so that the mixture stays meaty like lobster salad—and so I can eat the shrimp one by one straight from the fridge. If your shrimp salad actually makes it to the table, try it served in half an avocado, or place scoops in butter lettuce wraps and dab some Easiest Tartar Sauce (page 19) on top. It's a fantastic afternoon pick-me-up.

PREP TIME: 10 MINUTES

– ONE POT
– NO COOK
– 30 MINUTES
– 5 INGREDIENTS

3 dozen shrimp, cooked and peeled

¼ cup avocado oil

1 tablespoon chopped fresh cilantro

1 teaspoon cayenne

1 teaspoon garlic salt

1 teaspoon freshly ground black pepper

1 In a large bowl, mix together the shrimp, avocado oil, cilantro, cayenne, garlic salt, and pepper.

2 Serve immediately or store in an airtight container in the refrigerator for up to 5 days.

PER SERVING
Macronutrients: Fat 50%; Protein 48%; Carbs 2%
Calories: 165; Total Fat: 9g; Protein: 20g; Total Carbs: 1g; Fiber: 0g; Net Carbs: 1g

SALMON SALAD

— SERVES 6 —

I like to form servings of this salmon salad into a ball (similar to a cheese ball) and plate it with keto crackers or vegetables. It's perfect for book club or a cocktail party, maybe with some veggies for dipping. You could also serve it for lunch, in a lettuce cup with diced tomato and a little nondairy ranch dressing.

PREP TIME: 10 MINUTES

COOK TIME: 20 MINUTES

– 30 MINUTES

– 5 INGREDIENTS

1 garlic clove, unpeeled

4 (6-ounce) salmon fillets

4 ounces dairy-free cream cheese (such as Kite Hill)

2 teaspoons olive oil

2 teaspoons chopped fresh dill

1 teaspoon salt

1 Preheat the oven to 350°F.

2 Put the garlic clove in a small saucepan and cover with cold water. Bring to a boil and then remove from the heat. Let the garlic cool in the water.

3 Line a large rimmed baking sheet with parchment paper.

4 Arrange the salmon in a single layer on the prepared baking sheet and bake in the pre-heated oven for 20 minutes, until it is cooked through and flakes easily with a fork. Remove from the oven and let cool.

5 Once the garlic is cool, remove the peel and mince the clove.

6 Once the salmon is cool, use your hands to shred it into a small bowl. Add the cream cheese, olive oil, dill, salt, and garlic.

7 Stir together and serve immediately or store covered in the refrigerator for up to 5 days.

SIMPLIFY IT! If you have leftover Baked Salmon (page 93), this is a great way to repurpose it for another meal.

PER SERVING

Macronutrients: Fat 60%; Protein 36%; Carbs 4%

Calories: 291; Total Fat: 19g; Protein: 26g; Total Carbs: 4g; Fiber: 0g; Net Carbs: 4g

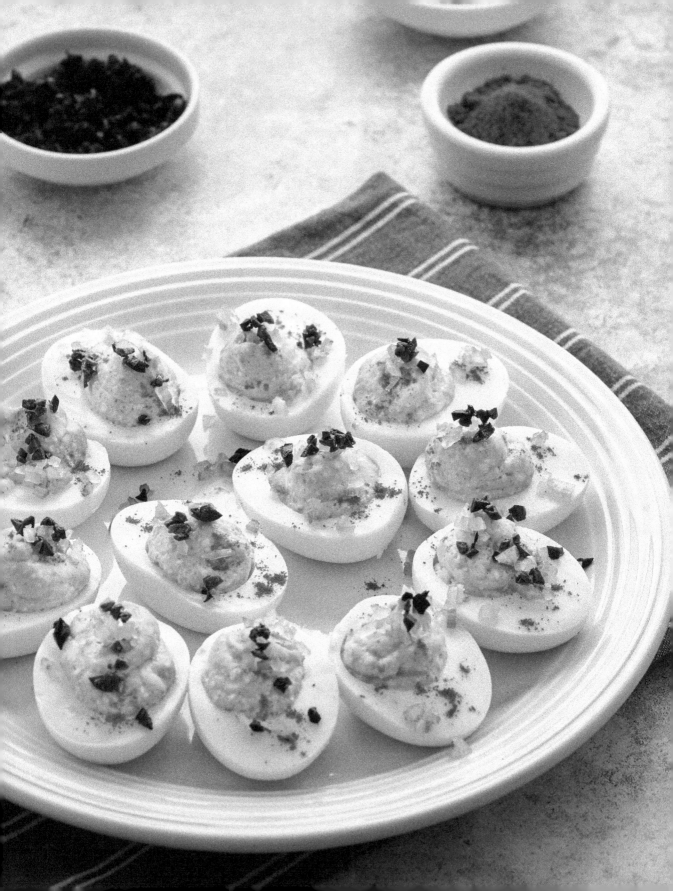

sides & snacks

Opposite: Deviled Eggs, page 68

GREEN BEAN AND MUSHROOM CASSEROLE

— SERVES 6 —

When I first started my dairy-free keto eating plan, there were certain foods that I missed all the way down to the bottom of my soul. The classic green bean casserole was one of those. I created this version one year for Thanksgiving, and now it makes regular appearances on our table all year long. It's got fresh green beans and mushrooms, a rich, creamy sauce, and a crunchy topping of slivered almonds. What more could you need?

PREP TIME: 15 MINUTES

COOK TIME: 1 HOUR

– ONE POT

2 tablespoons olive oil, divided

1 pound fresh green beans, trimmed and cut into 2- to 3-inch lengths

12 ounces mushrooms, sliced

1 onion, diced

1 shallot, diced

1 (14-ounce) can coconut milk

½ cup bone broth

3 tablespoons minced garlic

1 teaspoon salt

1 teaspoon freshly ground black pepper

½ cup slivered almonds

1 Preheat the oven to 350°F. Grease a 9-by-13-inch baking dish with 1 tablespoon of oil.

2 In the prepared baking dish, toss the green beans, mushrooms, onion, and shallot together with the remaining tablespoon of oil.

3 Pour the coconut milk and broth over the vegetables, and add the garlic, salt, and pepper. Stir gently to mix. Sprinkle the slivered almonds over the top.

4 Bake in the preheated oven for 1 hour, or until cooked through.

SUBSTITUTION TIP: For a vegetarian version, substitute vegetable broth for the bone broth.

PER SERVING

Macronutrients: Fat 72%; Protein 11%; Carbs 17%
Calories: 263; Total Fat: 21g; Protein: 7g; Total
Carbs: 15g; Fiber: 5g; Net Carbs: 10g

PROSCIUTTO-WRAPPED ASPARAGUS WITH LEMON-GARLIC DRESSING

— SERVES 6 —

This is what I like to call "company food": dishes that are stunning, tasty, and perfect for when we have friends over. This appetizer looks beautiful straight out of the oven. It's no-fuss, but the simple ingredients make it seem fancy. Use nice, plump asparagus spears if they're available, rather than the pencil-thin ones. If you don't have prosciutto, wrap the asparagus bundles with strips of bacon.

PREP TIME: 10 MINUTES

COOK TIME: 20 MINUTES

– ONE POT
– 30 MINUTES
– 5 INGREDIENTS

Oil, for greasing the baking sheet

12 slices prosciutto

36 fresh asparagus spears, trimmed

¼ cup Lemon-Garlic Dressing (page 16)

1 Preheat the oven to 350°F. Grease a large rimmed baking sheet.

2 Wrap 2 slices of prosciutto around 6 asparagus spears. Repeat with the remaining prosciutto and asparagus to form a total of 6 bundles.

3 Arrange the prosciutto-wrapped asparagus bundles on the baking sheet and pour the dressing over the top.

4 Bake in the preheated oven for 20 minutes. Serve hot.

INGREDIENT TIP: Asparagus can sometimes have woody ends. The best way to get rid of any woody bits is to hold the asparagus spear with one end in each hand and bend it until it snaps. It will snap right where the woody part ends and the tender stalk begins.

PER SERVING

Macronutrients: Fat 65%; Protein 29%; Carbs 6%
Calories: 448; Total Fat: 32g; Protein: 33g; Total Carbs: 5g; Fiber: 2g; Net Carbs: 3g

ROSEMARY AND GARLIC–ROASTED RADISHES

— SERVES 4 —

Radishes are really unsung heroes of the veggie world. They get relegated to garnish or salad filler, but they're so much more versatile than most people realize. When roasted, they develop a texture similar to a potato's, and the oven brings out a buttery flavor hiding beneath the sharp tang. Adding fresh herbs like rosemary makes them taste even more like your favorite roasted taters.

PREP TIME: 15 MINUTES

COOK TIME: 45 MINUTES

– ONE POT

– 5 INGREDIENTS

2 bunches radishes (about 24 radishes), quartered

¼ cup olive oil

2 tablespoons minced fresh rosemary

1½ teaspoons garlic salt

1 teaspoon freshly ground black pepper

1 Preheat the oven to 350ºF.

2 In a 9-by-13-inch baking dish, toss together the radishes, olive oil, rosemary, garlic salt, and pepper.

3 Bake in the preheated oven for 45 minutes. Serve hot.

PER SERVING

Macronutrients: Fat 85%; Protein 5%; Carbs 10%

Calories: 133; Total Fat: 13g; Protein: 1g; Total Carbs: 3g; Fiber: 1g; Net Carbs: 2g

CREAM CHEESE SAUSAGE DIP

— SERVES 8 —

Hot, cheesy dip with sausage is welcome on my table anytime, but especially during football season, when it feels like a party every weekend. This dip cooks in the slow cooker, which also allows you to keep it warm until the final seconds of the game. I like to serve it with raw vegetables for dipping.

PREP TIME: 5 MINUTES

COOK TIME: 8 HOURS

– ONE POT

– 5 INGREDIENTS

2 (10-ounce) cans diced tomatoes with green chiles

2 (8-ounce) containers dairy-free cream cheese (such as Kite Hill)

1 pound loose sausage

1 In a slow cooker, combine the tomatoes, cream cheese, and sausage, and stir to mix.

2 Cover and cook for 8 hours on low.

INGREDIENT TIP: If you brown the sausage in a skillet before adding it to the slow cooker with the other ingredients, you can cut the cooking time down to 4 hours on low.

PER SERVING
Macronutrients: Fat 80%; Protein 14%; Carbs 6%
Calories: 360; Total Fat: 32g; Protein: 13g; Total Carbs: 5g; Fiber: 0g; Net Carbs: 5g

TURNIPS AU GRATIN

— SERVES 8 —

Don't underestimate the humble turnip; it makes a great potato substitute. In this recipe, the turnips are sliced thin and layered with dairy-free cream cheese, yielding an indulgent yet keto-friendly dish that's bursting with flavor (jalapeño adds a kick). My husband's exact words were "Babe, this is the best thing you've ever made." Add some sausage to make it a one-dish dinner, or just serve the turnips on their own. You'll never miss the cheese.

PREP TIME: 15 MINUTES

COOK TIME: 1 HOUR

3 medium turnips, very thinly sliced

2 teaspoons freshly ground black pepper

1 teaspoon salt

1 (8-ounce) container dairy-free cream cheese (such as Kite Hill)

4 cups bone broth

1 jalapeño pepper, sliced into thin rings

¾ cup bacon bits

2 tablespoons dried or fresh chives

1 Preheat the oven to 350°F.

2 Arrange the turnip slices overlapping each other to cover the bottom of a 9-by-13-inch baking dish. Season with the pepper and salt.

3 In a small bowl, whisk together the cream cheese and bone broth until blended. Pour the mixture over the turnips. Arrange the jalapeño slices on top. Bake in the preheated oven for 1 hour.

4 Sprinkle the bacon bits and chives over the top and serve hot.

SUBSTITUTION TIP: For a vegetarian version, substitute vegetable broth for the bone broth.

PER SERVING

Macronutrients: Fat 48%; Protein 34%; Carbs 18%

Calories: 190; Total Fat: 10g; Protein: 16g; Total Carbs: 9g; Fiber: 2g; Net Carbs: 7g

TURNIP FRIES

— SERVES 4 —

You don't have to miss out on French fries just because you're eating keto. These turnip fries may sound odd, but they are so, so good. Eat them with Beef Liver Burgers (page 118) to satisfy all your burger-and-fries cravings. Your own kitchen will become your new favorite (keto-friendly) fast-food joint.

PREP TIME: 20 MINUTES

COOK TIME: 1 HOUR

– 5 INGREDIENTS

1 teaspoon salt

1 teaspoon freshly ground black pepper

1 teaspoon cayenne

2 large turnips, cut into ¼-inch-wide sticks

6 tablespoons grapeseed oil

1 Preheat the oven to 375°F. Line a baking sheet with parchment paper.

2 In a large bowl, stir together the salt, pepper, and cayenne. Add the turnips and olive oil, and toss to coat well.

3 Transfer the turnips to the prepared baking sheet and bake in the preheated oven for 1 hour, or until browned and crisp. Serve hot.

PER SERVING

Macronutrients: Fat 88%; Protein 3%; Carbs 9%

Calories: 221; Total Fat: 21g; Protein: 1g; Total Carbs: 6g; Fiber: 2g; Net Carbs: 4g

SIGNATURE BEEF JERKY

— MAKES ABOUT 30 PIECES —

Beef jerky is a great grab-and-go snack that is low in carbs and full of protein. Store-bought versions often have a lot of sugar, though, and they can be expensive. This keto-friendly version is easy to make at home and has become one of my favorite go-to snacks to have around at all times. The recipe makes a lot, and it stores well in the refrigerator.

PREP TIME: 20 MINUTES

COOK TIME: 3 HOURS

– 5 INGREDIENTS

2 tablespoons olive oil

1 tablespoon red pepper flakes

1½ teaspoons minced garlic

1 teaspoon salt

1 teaspoon freshly ground pepper

1 teaspoon dried mustard

1 pound precut (1½-inch-wide) sirloin steak strips

1 Preheat the oven to 225ºF.

2 Line a large baking sheet with parchment paper or a silicone baking mat.

3 In a large bowl, stir together the olive oil, red pepper flakes, garlic, salt, pepper, and dried mustard. Add the steak strips and use your hands to toss them in the oil mixture to coat thoroughly.

4 Arrange the steak strips in a single layer on the prepared baking sheet.

5 Bake in the preheated oven for 3 hours, or until the steak is dry and wrinkled.

6 Store the jerky in an airtight container in the refrigerator for up to 10 days.

VARIATION TIP: You may want to experiment a bit with the cooking time, depending on how you like your jerky. Three hours delivers the perfect texture for me, but you might prefer your jerky a little more or less dry.

PER SERVING (6 PIECES)
Macronutrients: Fat 49%; Protein 49%; Carbs 2%
Calories: 148; Total Fat: 8g; Protein: 18g; Total Carbs: 1g; Fiber: 0g; Net Carbs: 1g

SALAMI, DILL PICKLE, AND CREAM CHEESE TACOS

— SERVES 4 —

These "tacos" are hands down my favorite fast-food-type lunch, but so much better than anything you could order at a drive-through. It ticks all the boxes for me: easy, delicious, and colorful on the plate. I eat these at least once a week; my favorite part is the dill pickles (they should be their own food group, if you ask me), but feel free to omit them if they're not to your taste.

PREP TIME: 10 MINUTES

– ONE POT
– NO COOK
– 30 MINUTES
– 5 INGREDIENTS

8 slices salami (I like Applegate Farms)

4 whole kosher dill pickles, cut into thin rounds

2 tablespoons dairy-free cream cheese (like Kite Hill)

1 On a small plate, stack the salami slices in pairs to make four "shells."

2 Spread the cream cheese on each salami stack, then add the pickles.

3 Fold each salami stack like a taco and eat.

SUBSTITUTION TIP: You can replace cream cheese with sugar-free mayonnaise, depending on what you have in the kitchen.

PER SERVING
Macronutrients: Fat 73%; Protein 17%; Carbs 10%
Calories: 161; Total Fat: 13g; Protein: 7g; Total Carbs: 4g; Fiber: 0g; Net Carbs: 4g

MUSHROOM PIZZA BITES

— MAKES 24 BITES —

I love serving warm appetizers for a party or whenever I have guests.
Everyone loves pizza, and these upgraded pizza bites are a nice change of
pace from the usual forbidden party foods like chips and cheese. They make
a fun presentation, too, with the fixings packed into the mushroom tops.

PREP TIME: 10 MINUTES

COOK TIME: 7 MINUTES

− ONE POT

− 30 MINUTES

2 tablespoons olive oil, plus more for greasing the baking sheet

24 whole mushrooms, stemmed

½ cup low-carb marinara sauce (such as Rao's Homemade)

24 slices pepperoni

1 tablespoon dried oregano

1 tablespoon dried basil

1 teaspoon garlic salt

1 Preheat the broiler on low. Grease a large baking sheet with oil.

2 Arrange the mushrooms in a single layer on the prepared baking sheet, upside down so that they form little "bowls."

3 Add a spoonful of sauce to the center of each mushroom, then top it with a pepperoni slice.

4 Sprinkle the oregano, basil, and garlic salt over the mushrooms, then drizzle them with the olive oil.

5 Cook under the broiler for 5 to 7 minutes, or until the sauce is bubbling and the pepperoni begins to turn crisp and brown around the edges.

SIMPLIFY IT! To minimize cleanup, you can line the baking sheet with aluminum foil, but whatever you do, don't use parchment paper under the broiler, as it will catch fire. (Ask me how I know!)

PER SERVING (4 BITES)
Macronutrients: Fat 74%; Protein 14%; Carbs 12%
Calories: 101; Total Fat: 8g; Protein: 4g; Total
Carbs: 4g; Fiber: 1g; Net Carbs: 3g

NO-FAIL HARD-BOILED EGGS

— MAKES 12 EGGS —

Hard-boiled eggs are a big part of my dairy-free keto diet. And I know what you're thinking: *It's not like it's difficult to boil an egg, right?* The thing is, people ask me all the time what method I recommend. So here's my perfect, no-fail egg-boiling technique.

PREP TIME: 2 MINUTES

COOK TIME: 15 MINUTES

– ONE POT

– 30 MINUTES

– 5 INGREDIENTS

12 large eggs

1 Place the eggs in a medium saucepan and fill it halfway with water so that the eggs are submerged.

2 Bring to a boil. As soon as the water boils, set your timer for 7 minutes. When the timer beeps, turn off the burner but leave the pot on the stovetop. Let sit for 7 more minutes. Drain.

3 Peel the eggs under warm running water.

PER SERVING (1 EGG)

Macronutrients: Fat 63%; Protein 35%; Carbs 2%

Calories: 71; Total Fat: 5g; Protein: 6g; Total Carbs: 0g; Fiber: 0g; Net Carbs: 0g

DEVILED EGGS

— MAKES 12 HALVES —

I so love a good deviled egg. Lucky for me, they're a great dairy-free keto snack. They're easy to make and contain lots of healthy fat. You can get fancy with the toppings if you want, but I usually just keep them simple.

PREP TIME: 20 MINUTES

– NO COOK

– 5 INGREDIENTS

6 No-Fail Hard-Boiled Eggs (page 67), peeled

¾ cup sugar-free mayonnaise (such as Primal Kitchen)

2 teaspoons Swerve granular (or other granulated alternative sweetener)

1 teaspoon yellow mustard

1 teaspoon paprika

1 Halve the eggs lengthwise and create egg-white "bowls" by using a spoon to gently scoop out the yolks. Transfer the yolks to a small mixing bowl.

2 Add the mayonnaise, sweetener, and mustard to the yolks. Stir to mix well.

3 Arrange the egg whites in a small baking dish, with the "bowl" side facing up. Spoon the yolk mixture into the center of the eggs. Sprinkle with the paprika.

4 Serve immediately or cover and refrigerate for up to 2 days.

VARIATION TIP: Try topping your deviled eggs with minced celery, black olives, cracked pepper-corns, or your favorite hot sauce.

PER SERVING (2 HALVES)
Macronutrients: Fat 89%; Protein 8%; Carbs 3%
Calories: 293; Total Fat: 29g; Protein: 6g; Total
Carbs: 2g; Fiber: 0g; Net Carbs: 2g; Erythritol 0.5g

CREAMED SPINACH

— SERVES 4 —

Traditional creamed spinach—cooked with butter and heavy cream—is
so rich and dreamy. For this version, I use dairy-free cream cheese, and it
turns out every bit as luxurious. I like to serve this spinach as a side with my
Lemon-Garlic Pork Tenderloin with Radishes and Green Pepper (page 129).

PREP TIME: 5 MINUTES

COOK TIME: 10 MINUTES

– ONE POT
– 30 MINUTES
– 5 INGREDIENTS

2 tablespoons olive oil

1 onion, diced

1 (12-ounce) bag spinach

1 teaspoon minced garlic

1 (8-ounce) container dairy-free
cream cheese (such as Kite Hill)

Salt

Freshly ground black pepper

1 Heat the oil in a skillet over medium-high
heat. Add the onion and cook, stirring frequently, until softened, about 5 minutes.
Add the spinach and garlic and cook, stirring
frequently, until the spinach is wilted, about
2 minutes.

2 Reduce the heat to low and stir in the cream
cheese. Cook, stirring, until the cream cheese
is completely melted and the mixture is well
combined, about 2 minutes.

3 Season with salt and pepper to taste, and
serve immediately.

SUBSTITUTION TIP: You can make this dish
with other greens like kale or chard; just add a
few minutes to the cooking time.

PER SERVING
Macronutrients: Fat 76%; Protein 12%; Carbs 12%
Calories: 249; Total Fat: 21g; Protein: 7g; Total
Carbs: 8g; Fiber: 2g; Net Carbs: 6g

CAULIFLOWER MASH

— SERVES 5 —

Mashed cauliflower is a great stand-in for mashed potatoes—I've even come to like it better than the original because it's a bit lighter and has more flavor. I use the cream from the top of a can of coconut milk because it has the highest fat content and adds great texture, making the dish ultra-creamy and decadent.

PREP TIME: 20 MINUTES

COOK TIME: 20 MINUTES

– 5 INGREDIENTS

1 head cauliflower, cut into large chunks

½ can coconut milk (cream from the top only)

⅓ cup olive oil

1½ teaspoons freshly ground black pepper

1 teaspoon salt

½ teaspoon cayenne

1 teaspoon chopped fresh chives

¼ cup bacon bits

1 Preheat the oven to 350°F.

2 In a large pot, cover the cauliflower with water and bring to a boil until softened.

3 Transfer the cauliflower to a blender and add the coconut milk cream, olive oil, pepper, salt, and cayenne. Blend until smooth. Pour the mixture into a 9-inch square baking dish and bake for 20 minutes, or until the top is lightly browned.

4 Serve hot, topped with the fresh chives and bacon bits.

SUBSTITUTION TIP: In place of a head of cauliflower, you can also use a 12-ounce bag of riced cauliflower. Instead of boiling it, just heat it in the microwave according to the package directions, then continue with the rest of the recipe.

PER SERVING

Macronutrients: Fat 85%; Protein 8%; Carbs 7%
Calories: 265; Total Fat: 26g; Protein: 5g; Total Carbs: 5g; Fiber: 2g; Net Carbs: 3g

BRUSSELS SPROUTS WITH BACON

— SERVES 4 —

I like to have something green on every dinner plate, and these are an easy throw-in-the-oven side to make any dinner pop. Shave the Brussels sprouts thin for a crunchier dish; they're perfect however you slice them.

PREP TIME: 10 MINUTES

COOK TIME: 50 MINUTES

– ONE POT

– 5 INGREDIENTS

2 bunches Brussels sprouts (24 to 30), trimmed and halved

6 strips uncooked bacon, diced

5 tablespoons olive oil

1 tablespoon minced garlic

1 teaspoon salt

1 teaspoon freshly ground black pepper

1 Preheat the oven to 350°F.

2 In a 9-by-13-inch baking dish, toss the Brussels sprouts with the bacon and olive oil.

3 Stir in the garlic, salt, and pepper.

4 Bake for 50 minutes, or until the Brussels sprouts are tender.

SUBSTITUTION TIP: To make this vegetarian, omit the bacon. Add 2 diced turnips along with the Brussels sprouts.

PER SERVING

Macronutrients: Fat 82%; Protein 8%; Carbs 10%

Calories: 394; Total Fat: 36g; Protein: 9g; Total Carbs: 11g; Fiber: 4g; Net Carbs: 7g

SLOW-COOKER LI'L SMOKIES

— MAKES 48 MINI HOT DOGS —

I love throwing these cute little dogs in the slow cooker for an easy hot appetizer when we're entertaining. It turns out that just about everyone loves mini hot dogs, and cooking them in a quick keto "barbecue" sauce makes them irresistible. I serve them right in the slow cooker (set to Keep Warm), with toothpicks for easy pickup.

PREP TIME: 5 MINUTES

COOK TIME: 4 HOURS

– ONE POT

– 5 INGREDIENTS

2 (8-ounce) packages mini hot dogs (I love the ones from Teton Waters Ranch)

¼ cup sugar-free ketchup (such as Primal Kitchen)

¼ cup white vinegar

3 tablespoons whole-grain mustard

1 teaspoon Swerve granular (or other granulated alternative sweetener)

1 In a slow cooker, combine the mini hot dogs, ketchup, white vinegar, mustard, and sweetener.

2 Cover and cook on low for 4 hours.

PER SERVING (4 MINI HOT DOGS)
Macronutrients: Fat 82%; Protein 14%; Carbs 4%
Calories: 119; Total Fat: 11g; Protein: 4g; Total Carbs: 1g; Fiber: 0g; Net Carbs: 1g; Erythritol 0.5g

CUCUMBER-SALAMI STACKS

— MAKES 24 STACKS —

I love making these little bites to have for lunch or take to a friend's house for an easy hors d'oeuvre. It's trick food (no one has to know it's keto) that looks great and will be a hit with everyone.

PREP TIME: 5 MINUTES

– ONE POT
– NO COOK
– 30 MINUTES
– 5 INGREDIENTS

2 large cucumbers, sliced into about 24 thick rounds

24 (or however many cucumber slices you have) bite-size salami pieces

½ cup dairy-free cream cheese (such as Kite Hill)

24 cherry or grape tomatoes

On top of each cucumber slice, place a piece of salami and top it with about 1 teaspoon of cream cheese and a cherry tomato. Add a toothpick to each stack to hold it together.

PER SERVING (4 STACKS)

Macronutrients: Fat 81%; Protein 13%; Carbs 6%
Calories: 313; Total Fat: 28g; Protein: 13g; Total Carbs: 7g; Fiber: 2g; Net Carbs: 5g

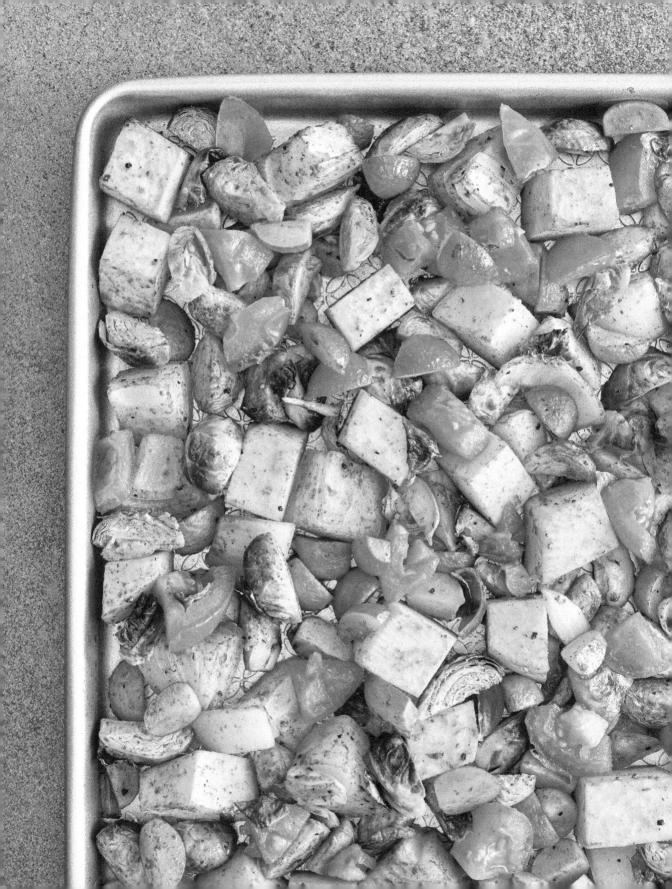

CHAPTER 6

vegetarian & vegan mains

Opposite: Vegetable Bake with Cayenne Pepper, page 76

VEGETABLE BAKE WITH CAYENNE PEPPER

— SERVES 12 —

I love to make a big pan of baked or roasted vegetables at the beginning of the week. I eat them all week long, as a side dish with roasted or grilled meats, topped with fried eggs for a quick breakfast-for-dinner, or on their own as a light meal. Brussels sprouts are one of my favorite vegetables for this kind of dish, because they're sturdy enough to hold up during the long bake without turning mushy. Their leafy edges tend to brown and crisp up, giving the dish delicious texture.

PREP TIME: 20 MINUTES

COOK TIME: 1 HOUR

– ONE POT

1 bunch Brussels sprouts (about 20), diced

1 tomato, diced

1 bunch radishes (about 12), diced

1 onion, diced

2 turnips, diced

6 tablespoons olive oil

¼ cup cayenne

2 teaspoons salt

1 teaspoon freshly ground black pepper

1 Preheat the oven to 400°F.

2 Toss the Brussels sprouts, tomato, radishes, onion, and turnips together on a large rimmed baking sheet. Add the olive oil and toss to coat well. Season with the cayenne, salt, and pepper.

3 Bake in the preheated oven for 1 hour, or until the vegetables are browned and crisp. Store covered in the refrigerator for up to 1 week.

SUBSTITUTION TIP: Make this dish your own by substituting different vegetables. Broccoli, cauliflower, or asparagus could all take the place of the Brussels sprouts—or just add them to the mix. You may need to adjust the cooking time a bit when using more delicate vegetables.

PER SERVING

Macronutrients: Fat 66%; Protein 9%; Carbs 25%

Calories: 95; Total Fat: 7g; Protein: 2g; Total Carbs: 6g; Fiber: 2g; Net Carbs: 4g

CAULIFLOWER STEAKS

— SERVES 4 —

Cauliflower gets used a lot in keto recipes because it makes such a great substitute for starchy base ingredients like potatoes, rice, and pasta. Here it shines as the star of the dish—sliced into "steaks," basted with a mustard marinade, and roasted until golden brown. Serve these alongside a hearty salad, like Broccoli Salad (page 47) or Wedge Salad with Ranch Dressing (page 49).

PREP TIME: 10 MINUTES

COOK TIME: 25 MINUTES

– 5 INGREDIENTS

2 tablespoons olive oil, plus more for greasing the baking sheet

2 tablespoons whole-grain mustard

1 teaspoon garlic salt

1 teaspoon capers

1 head cauliflower, sliced into 2 (¾-inch-wide) "steaks"

1 Preheat the oven to 400°F. Grease a large baking sheet.

2 In a small bowl, stir together the mustard, oil, garlic salt, and capers.

3 Arrange the cauliflower steaks on the prepared baking sheet in a single layer and then pour the mustard mixture over the top, spreading it to coat evenly.

4 Bake in the preheated oven for 20 minutes.

5 Turn the oven to broil and cook the steaks under the broiler for about 5 minutes, or until the tops of the steaks are nicely browned.

PER SERVING

Macronutrients: Fat 60%; Protein 10%; Carbs 30%
Calories: 120; Total Fat: 8g; Protein: 3g; Total
Carbs: 9g; Fiber: 3g; Net Carbs: 6g

VARIATION TIP: Serve with Lemon-Garlic Dressing (page 16) for a nice complement to the mustard marinade. The added sauce will adjust your macros, increasing fat and decreasing carbs.

LEMON-GARLIC KALE WITH RADISHES AND SUNFLOWER SEEDS

— SERVES 4 —

This unexpected combination—warm roasted kale and radishes, savory marinade, and lots of garlic, plus the crunch of sunflower seeds—is divine. It looks beautiful on the table, too, so it's a great dish for company.

PREP TIME: 15 MINUTES

COOK TIME: 1 HOUR

– ONE POT

– 5 INGREDIENTS

Oil, for greasing the baking sheet

1 bunch radishes (about 12), diced

½ teaspoon salt

½ teaspoon freshly ground black pepper

1 (16-ounce) bag kale, chopped

5 tablespoons Lemon-Garlic Dressing (page 16)

¼ cup raw, salted sunflower seeds

2 tablespoons minced garlic

1 Preheat the oven to 400°F. Grease a large rimmed baking sheet with oil.

2 Arrange the diced radishes in a single layer on the prepared baking sheet and season with the salt and pepper.

3 Bake in the preheated oven for 40 minutes.

4 Remove the baking sheet from the oven and add the kale, dressing, sunflower seeds, and garlic. Toss to combine.

5 Return the baking sheet to the oven and continue to cook for 20 minutes, or until the kale is crunchy.

SUBSTITUTION TIP: If kale isn't your go-to, you can swap in broccoli, broccoli rabe, or green beans instead. Also try slivered almonds in place of the sunflower seeds.

PER SERVING
Macronutrients: Fat 64%; Protein 8%; Carbs 28%
Calories: 198; Total Fat: 14g; Protein: 4g; Total Carbs: 14g; Fiber: 2g; Net Carbs: 12g

RADISHES WITH OLIVES, CAPERS, AND TOMATO SAUCE

— SERVES 5 —

This pasta-esque dish is destined to become part of your regular rotation. The radishes are a great noodle substitute, thanks to their firm texture and ability to take on any flavor. The savory, briny tomato sauce will have everyone reaching for seconds—and volunteering to clean the kitchen just to just grab those last few morsels.

PREP TIME: 15 MINUTES

COOK TIME: 1 HOUR

– 5 INGREDIENTS

2 bunches radishes (about 24), quartered

2 teaspoons salt

1 teaspoon freshly ground black pepper

6 tablespoons olive oil, divided

2 (14.5-ounce) cans diced tomatoes, with their juices

3 ounces black olives, sliced

3 tablespoons capers

1 Preheat the oven to 375°F.

2 In a 9-inch square baking dish, toss the radishes with the salt, pepper, and 3 tablespoons of olive oil. Bake, uncovered, in the preheated oven for 1 hour.

3 While the radishes bake, in a medium saucepan, combine the tomatoes (with their juices), olives, capers, and the remaining 3 tablespoons of olive oil. Bring to a simmer over medium-high heat, then reduce the heat to low and simmer, stirring occasionally, for 45 minutes, or until the sauce thickens and the flavors are well combined.

4 Remove the radishes from the oven and pour the sauce over the top. Serve immediately or store in an airtight container in the refrigerator for up to 1 week.

PER SERVING
Macronutrients: Fat 88%; Protein 2%; Carbs 10%
Calories: 195; Total Fat: 19g; Protein: 1g; Total Carbs: 5g; Fiber: 2g; Net Carbs: 3g

CAULIFLOWER AND ONION SOUFFLÉS

— SERVES 6 —

The word *soufflé* makes any recipe sound decidedly gourmet. It also makes it sound a bit intimidating for all but the most seasoned cooks. But you'll be shocked to discover how easy this recipe is. The individual soufflés are light and fluffy, but packed with healthy cauliflower.

PREP TIME: 10 MINUTES

COOK TIME: 30 MINUTES

– 5 INGREDIENTS

Oil, for greasing the soufflé dishes

1 recipe Cauliflower Mash (page 70)

2 large eggs, beaten

1 onion, finely chopped

1 tablespoon cayenne

1 tablespoon dried chives

1 Preheat the oven to 375°F. Grease 6 (6-ounce) soufflé dishes or ramekins with oil.

2 In a large bowl, whisk together the Cauliflower Mash, eggs, onion, cayenne, and chives.

3 Spoon the mixture into the prepared soufflé dishes and bake for 30 minutes, or until puffed and golden brown on top.

4 Serve hot.

PER SERVING

Macronutrients: Fat 82%; Protein 9%; Carbs 9%

Calories: 308; Total Fat: 28g; Protein: 7g; Total Carbs: 7g; Fiber: 3g; Net Carbs: 4g

CASHEW VEGETABLES OVER CAULIFLOWER RICE

— SERVES 6 —

Cashews add a welcome soft crunch and a rich earthiness to a vegetarian stir-fry. This is a full meal in itself, but I also like to stuff it into lettuce cups and drizzle with a little chili oil as an appetizer or light lunch.

PREP TIME: 10 MINUTES

COOK TIME: 25 MINUTES

– ONE POT

5 tablespoons sesame oil, divided

1 onion, chopped

8 ounces mushrooms, sliced

1 green bell pepper, seeded and chopped

1 red bell pepper, seeded and chopped

½ cup raw cashews

¼ cup coconut aminos

1 teaspoon garlic salt

1 (12-ounce) bag riced cauliflower, cooked according to the package directions

1 Heat 2 tablespoons of sesame oil in a skillet over medium-high heat. Add the onion and cook, stirring frequently, until softened, about 5 minutes.

2 Add the remaining 3 tablespoons of sesame oil, followed by the mushrooms, green bell pepper, red bell pepper, cashews, coconut aminos, and garlic salt. Cook for 20 minutes, or until vegetables are tender.

3 Serve the stir-fried vegetables hot over the cauliflower rice.

INGREDIENT TIP: Coconut aminos is a seasoning sauce made from coconut blossom sap and sea salt. It's like soy sauce, but lower in sodium, soy-free, gluten-free, vegan, and, of course, keto friendly.

PER SERVING

Macronutrients: Fat 66%; Protein 10%; Carbs 24%

Calories: 177; Total Fat: 13g; Protein: 4g; Total Carbs: 11g; Fiber: 4g; Net Carbs: 7g

EGGPLANT MARINARA

— SERVES 4 —

Eggplant is a real workhorse ingredient. It takes on a "meaty" texture when cooked, and it's also surprisingly versatile. I use keto-friendly almond flour in place of bread crumbs to coat the cutlets, and then top them with zesty marinara sauce.

PREP TIME: 20 MINUTES

COOK TIME: 1 HOUR

½ cup almond flour

1 teaspoon salt

1 teaspoon minced garlic

1 teaspoon onion powder

2 large eggs, lightly beaten

6 tablespoons olive oil

1 eggplant, sliced into ⅓-inch-thick rounds

1 cup sliced mushrooms

1 (10-ounce) bag spinach

1 (8-ounces) container dairy-free cream cheese (such as Kite Hill)

1 (24-ounce) jar low-carb marinara sauce (like Rao's Homemade)

1 Preheat the oven to 350°F.

2 In a medium bowl, mix together the almond flour, salt, garlic, and onion powder.

3 In another bowl, beat the eggs for dipping.

4 Heat the oil in a large skillet over medium-high heat.

5 One at a time, dip the eggplant slices, first in the eggs and then in the flour mixture, turning to coat. Transfer to the skillet and cook for 2 to 3 minutes per side, until golden brown.

6 Once the eggplant slices are browned, arrange them in a single layer in a large baking dish. When the bottom of the baking dish is covered, add layers of mushrooms, spinach, and cream cheese. Top with a second layer of browned eggplant, mushrooms, spinach, and cream cheese. Continue making layers until you run out of ingredients.

7 Pour the marinara sauce over the top of the layers.

8 Bake in the preheated oven for 40 minutes, or until the sauce is bubbling.

INGREDIENT TIP: If you find eggplant too bitter, salt your eggplant slices generously and let them sit on a paper towel–lined baking sheet for 30 minutes. Blot the salt and condensation from the slices with paper towels before coating them with the egg-and-flour mixture.

PER SERVING

Macronutrients: Fat 71%; Protein 12%; Carbs 17%
Calories: 495; Total Fat: 39g; Protein: 14g; Total Carbs: 22g; Fiber: 11g; Net Carbs: 11g

CREAM CHEESE–STUFFED MUSHROOMS

— SERVES 4 —

Portobello mushrooms are full of umami flavor, which is why they're such a great ingredient to use in meatless cooking. In this recipe, they're filled with a savory mixture of dairy-free cream cheese, capers, and chives, making for a satisfying main dish or a substantial side.

PREP TIME: 10 MINUTES

COOK TIME: 20 MINUTES

– 30 MINUTES

– 5 INGREDIENTS

¼ cup olive oil, plus more for greasing the baking sheet

4 portobello mushroom caps, stemmed

½ cup dairy-free cream cheese (such as Kite Hill)

2 tablespoons chopped fresh chives

4 teaspoons capers (optional)

1 teaspoon salt

1 teaspoon freshly ground black pepper

1 Preheat the oven to 350°F. Grease a baking sheet with oil.

2 Arrange the mushroom caps on the prepared baking sheet, underside-up.

3 In a small bowl, stir together the cream cheese, chives, and capers (if using).

4 Drizzle 1 tablespoon of olive oil over each mushroom cap. Spread about 2 tablespoons of the cream cheese mixture over each. Season with the salt and pepper.

5 Bake in the preheated oven for 20 minutes, or until the cream cheese is melted and bubbling.

SIMPLIFY IT! To make this recipe even easier, use a chive- or garlic-and-herb-flavored dairy-free cream cheese, like the Kite Hill Chive Cream Cheese style spread.

PER SERVING

Macronutrients: Fat 82%; Protein 9%; Carbs 9%
Calories: 295; Total Fat: 27g; Protein: 6g; Total Carbs: 7g; Fiber: 2g; Net Carbs: 5g

BUFFALO "MAC-AND-CHEESE" BAKE

— SERVES 8 —

How's this for a twist on a classic: a mac-and-cheese bake with no mac, no cheese, and an extra-spicy kick. Cauliflower, once again, takes on the noodle role, and nondairy alternatives like nutritional yeast and coconut milk do the rest of the work. Each bite is better than the last, especially with a tangy, creamy Buffalo-style sauce that will make you forget all about tradition.

PREP TIME: 20 MINUTES

COOK TIME: 1 HOUR

2 tablespoons olive oil, plus more for greasing the baking dish

2 (8-ounce) containers dairy-free cream cheese (such as Kite Hill)

2 pounds uncooked riced cauliflower

1 onion, diced

¾ cup hot wing sauce (such as Frank's RedHot)

½ cup canned coconut milk (or nut milk)

2 tablespoons minced garlic

2 tablespoons nutritional yeast

1 teaspoon salt

1 teaspoon freshly ground black pepper

3 tablespoons chopped fresh chives

1 Preheat the oven to 400°F. Grease a 9-by-13-inch baking dish.

2 In a large microwave-safe bowl, microwave the cream cheese on high for 1 minute to melt.

3 Into the bowl with the cream cheese, stir the cauliflower, onion, hot sauce, coconut milk (or nut milk), garlic, nutritional yeast, salt, and pepper. Mix well.

4 Transfer the mixture to the prepared baking dish. Drizzle the olive oil over the top.

5 Cook in the preheated oven for 1 hour, or until bubbly.

6 Serve hot, garnished with the chives.

PER SERVING

Macronutrients: Fat 70%; Protein 13%; Carbs 17%
Calories: 282; Total Fat: 22g; Protein: 9g; Total
Carbs: 12g; Fiber: 5g; Net Carbs: 7g

CAULIFLOWER BUFFALO WINGS

— SERVES 4 —

Traditional hot wings call for a number of non-keto, dairy-packed ingredients, like butter and breading, for starters. And it's certainly not vegetarian friendly. But you don't have to give up on the greatest party food known to humankind. If you love the flavors but want to skip the meat, dairy, and high carbs of the original, this dish is a dream come true. It's incredibly simple and super satisfying.

PREP TIME: 10 MINUTES

COOK TIME: 30 MINUTES

– 5 INGREDIENTS

1 head cauliflower, chopped into florets

1 onion, diced

1 (12-ounce) bottle hot wing sauce (such as Frank's RedHot)

3 tablespoons olive oil

2 tablespoons chopped fresh chives, for garnish

1 Preheat the oven to 425°F.

2 In a large bowl, combine the cauliflower, onion, wing sauce, and oil. Toss to coat the cauliflower evenly.

3 Arrange the cauliflower on a baking sheet in a single layer, with space in between the pieces if possible.

4 Bake in the preheated oven for 30 minutes, or until the cauliflower is crispy on the edges and golden brown.

5 Serve hot, garnished with the chives.

SERVING TIP: Serve these crunchy morsels with a dairy-free, keto-friendly ranch dressing (I like Primal Kitchen's) for dipping.

PER SERVING

Macronutrients: Fat 76%; Protein 6%; Carbs 18%
Calories: 131; Total Fat: 11g; Protein: 2g; Total Carbs: 6g; Fiber: 3g; Net Carbs: 3g

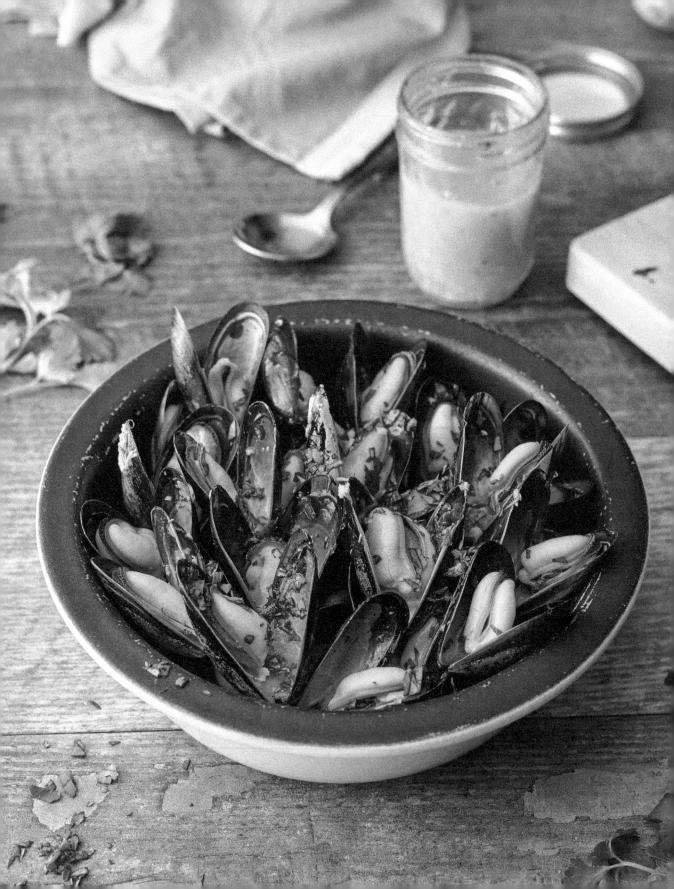

seafood

Opposite: Mussels with Lemon-Garlic Sauce and Parsley, page 95

COCONUT SHRIMP

— SERVES 4 —

Coconut is full of healthy fats; in this recipe, the crunchy coating contrasts nicely with the plump, tender shrimp. These make a great entrée, or you can leave the tails on the shrimp and serve them as finger food at your next party.

PREP TIME: 20 MINUTES

COOK TIME: 30 MINUTES

Avocado oil spray (or other cooking oil spray)

3 large egg whites

1 teaspoon cayenne

1 teaspoon garlic salt

1 teaspoon freshly ground black pepper

½ teaspoon Swerve granular (or other granulated alternative sweetener)

1 cup unsweetened shredded coconut

24 (or so) raw shrimp, peeled

1 Preheat the oven to 350°F. Spray a large baking sheet with the avocado oil spray.

2 In a small bowl, whisk together the egg whites, cayenne, garlic salt, pepper, and sweetener.

3 Put the shredded coconut in a separate bowl.

4 One at a time, dunk the shrimp first in the egg mixture and then in the coconut, turning to coat completely.

5 Arrange the coated shrimp on the prepared baking sheet in a single layer, with room in between. Once all the shrimp have been coated, spray them lightly with avocado oil spray.

6 Bake in the preheated oven for 30 minutes, or until the coconut is golden brown.

VARIATION TIP: To serve these with a spicy mayo for dipping, mix together ¼ cup sugar-free mayonnaise (such as Primal Kitchen) with chili paste or hot sauce to taste.

PER SERVING

Macronutrients: Fat 65%; Protein 22%; Carbs 13%
Calories: 223; Total Fat: 17g; Protein: 13g; Total Carbs: 7g; Fiber: 4g; Net Carbs: 3g; Erythritol 0.5g

BACON-WRAPPED SCALLOP CUPS

— SERVES 4 —

Bacon and scallops is a classic combination, and it's easy to see why: The salty, crisp bacon contrasts with the silky sweetness of the scallops so wonderfully. I love to serve these as an elegant hors d'oeuvre or with a colorful salad for a light entrée.

PREP TIME: 10 MINUTES

COOK TIME: 25 MINUTES

– ONE POT

– 5 INGREDIENTS

12 large sea scallops

6 strips bacon, halved to make 12 short strips

24 garlic cloves, peeled but left whole

5 tablespoons Lemon-Garlic Dressing (page 16)

1 Preheat the oven to 400°F.

2 Wrap each scallop with 1 piece of bacon. Use a toothpick to secure the bacon to the scallop. Arrange the wrapped scallops on a baking sheet.

3 Place 2 garlic cloves on top of each scallop, then top with a spoonful of the dressing.

4 Bake for 25 minutes, or until the bacon is browned and crisp.

PER SERVING

Macronutrients: Fat 63%; Protein 27%; Carbs 10%
Calories: 374; Total Fat: 26g; Protein: 26g; Total Carbs: 9g; Fiber: 0g; Net Carbs: 9g

SALMON PATTIES

— SERVES 5 —

My mom used to make salmon patties all the time when I was growing up, but I never appreciated how good they were. Back then, all I wanted was a peanut butter and jelly sandwich. (It was a classic example of not knowing how lucky I was.) When I went back to her recipe as an adult and adapted it for keto, it immediately took me back to my childhood—and I was finally able to appreciate my mom's good cooking. These are easy, too, using canned salmon you keep in the pantry. Serve them with some sugar-free ketchup or Easiest Tartar Sauce (page 19).

PREP TIME: 10 MINUTES

COOK TIME: 15 MINUTES

− 30 MINUTES

− 5 INGREDIENTS

2 (6-ounce) cans boneless salmon

1 large egg

1½ tablespoons chopped fresh dill

1 teaspoon salt

1 teaspoon freshly ground
black pepper

3 tablespoons olive oil

1 In a small mixing bowl, mix together the salmon, egg, dill, salt, and pepper. Form the salmon mixture into hamburger-size patties.

2 In a skillet over medium, heat the olive oil. Add the salmon patties to the skillet and cook for 3 to 4 minutes per side, or until golden brown and crisp. Serve hot.

VARIATION TIP: You can wrap the patties in lettuce leaves or other greens, or serve them atop a crisp green salad.

PER SERVING

Macronutrients: Fat 64%; Protein 34%; Carbs 2%
Calories: 198; Total Fat: 14g; Protein: 17g; Total Carbs: 1g; Fiber: 0g; Net Carbs: 1g

COUNTRY CLUB CRAB CAKES

— SERVES 4 —

I love a crab cake on a bed of greens. Top with my Lemon-Garlic Dressing (page 16) and a few blueberries and strawberries, and have your girlfriends over for a "fancy" lunch. Make sure to have my Lemon Squares (page 145) for dessert, too. There, I've just planned your next get-together!

PREP TIME: 10 MINUTES

COOK TIME: 20 MINUTES

− 30 MINUTES

− 5 INGREDIENTS

2 (6-ounce) cans crabmeat (or 12 ounces cooked crabmeat)

2 large eggs

2 tablespoons chopped fresh dill

1 teaspoon garlic salt

¼ cup olive oil

1 In a medium bowl, combine the crabmeat, eggs, dill, and garlic salt. Form the mixture into four patties.

2 In a medium skillet, heat the olive oil over medium heat. Cook the crab cakes for 3 to 4 minutes on each side, or until golden brown.

PER SERVING

Macronutrients: Fat 68%; Protein 30%; Carbs 2%
Calories: 212; Total Fat: 16g; Protein: 16g; Total Carbs: 1g; Fiber: 0g; Net Carbs: 1g

SHRIMP STIR-FRY

— SERVES 4 —

I love to keep frozen shrimp on hand because they're easy to defrost (under cold running water) and they cook up fast. If you've got a bag of shrimp in the freezer, it's likely you have everything you need to make this dish. It comes together in minutes, and tastes delicious—especially with a hit of hot chili sauce.

PREP TIME: 10 MINUTES

COOK TIME: 20 MINUTES

– ONE POT

– 30 MINUTES

1 (12-ounce) bag riced cauliflower

24 cooked and peeled shrimp

1 onion, diced

1 red bell pepper, chopped

2 cups chopped broccoli

¼ cup coconut aminos

¼ cup avocado oil

Chili sauce, for serving (optional)

1 In a large skillet, combine the cauliflower, shrimp, onion, bell pepper, broccoli, coconut aminos, and avocado oil. Cook, stirring occasionally, until all the flavors are combined, about 20 minutes.

2 Drizzle the chili sauce (if using) over the top and serve hot.

SUBSTITUTION TIP: You can substitute a meaty whitefish like cod for the shrimp—or even chicken, beef, or pork.

PER SERVING

Macronutrients: Fat 60%; Protein 20%; Carbs 20%
Calories: 231; Total Fat: 15g; Protein: 12g; Total Carbs: 12g; Fiber: 5g; Net Carbs: 7g

BAKED SALMON WITH LEMON AND MUSHROOMS

— SERVES 2 —

I love salmon for quick weeknight meals. It's such a meaty and flavorful fish, and you don't need to put a lot of work into it to turn it into a tasty dinner. It's also a great source of omega-3 fatty acids, those good fats that you want to eat more of. This recipe is so simple, and yet it still makes me feel like a hero in the kitchen.

PREP TIME: 10 MINUTES

COOK TIME: 30 MINUTES

– ONE POT

– 5 INGREDIENTS

2 (6-ounce) skin-on salmon fillets

1 onion, diced

8 ounces mushrooms, sliced

¼ cup olive oil

1 teaspoon salt

1 teaspoon freshly ground black pepper

4 lemon slices

1 Preheat the oven to 400°F.

2 Tear off 2 large squares of aluminum foil. Place a salmon fillet on each piece of foil and arrange the onion and mushrooms over and around the fish, dividing evenly.

3 Pour the olive oil over the fish, then season with the salt and pepper. Top each piece of fish with 2 lemon slices.

4 Wrap the foil up around the salmon and vegetables, leaving room inside the packet for heat to circulate, and bake for 30 minutes, or until the fish flakes easily with a fork. Serve hot.

PER SERVING

Macronutrients: Fat 70%; Protein 25%; Carbs 5%
Calories: 576; Total Fat: 44g; Protein: 37g; Total Carbs: 8g; Fiber: 3g; Net Carbs: 5g

PANFRIED SOFT-SHELL CRAB

— SERVES 2 —

The first time I cooked soft-shell crab, I was hesitant. But I love a challenge, and it turns out there's no need to be intimidated—it's easier than you might think. As soon as I fried a few of these for dinner, I was amazed by the simplicity of the process—and the incredibly tasty results. Now when soft-shell crabs are in season, you can find Brad and me camped out at the seafood counter in the grocery store, just waiting for them to appear. We love to eat them dunked in Easiest Tartar Sauce (page 19).

PREP TIME: 5 MINUTES

COOK TIME: 10 MINUTES

– 30 MINUTES

– 5 INGREDIENTS

½ cup olive oil

½ cup almond flour

1 teaspoon paprika

1 teaspoon garlic salt

1 teaspoon freshly ground black pepper

2 soft-shell crabs

1 Fill the bottom of a heavy skillet with the oil and heat over low heat.

2 While the oil is heating, in a medium bowl, mix together the almond flour, paprika, garlic salt, and pepper.

3 Dredge each crab in the flour mixture, coating both sides and shaking off any excess. Put the crabs into the hot oil in the skillet and cook for about 5 minutes per side, or until golden brown.

4 Serve hot.

INGREDIENT TIP: Soft-shell crabs are blue crabs (usually) that have shed their shells but haven't grown new, larger ones yet. They have the delicate, sweet flavor of crabmeat and are extra special because they can be eaten whole, making them much less work than regular crabs. They have a fairly short season, so you have to snap them up when you see them in the market.

PER SERVING

Macronutrients: Fat 61%; Protein 34%; Carbs 5%

Calories: 489; Total Fat: 33g; Protein: 42g; Total Carbs: 6g; Fiber: 2g; Net Carbs: 4g

MUSSELS WITH LEMON-GARLIC SAUCE AND PARSLEY

— SERVES 5 —

I used to think that cooking mussels was a laborious process best left to professional chefs. But then I discovered a well-kept secret: It's actually quite easy! I just cook them in a pot of boiling water and then drench them with my Lemon-Garlic Dressing (page 16). Is it wrong that I haven't let Brad in on the secret? I guess I just prefer for him to go on believing I'm a genius in the kitchen.

PREP TIME: 10 MINUTES

COOK TIME: 5 MINUTES

– ONE POT
– 30 MINUTES
– 5 INGREDIENTS

36 live mussels, scrubbed and debearded

1 tablespoon olive oil

6 tablespoons Lemon-Garlic Dressing (page 16)

2 tablespoons chopped fresh parsley, for garnish

1 Fill a stockpot halfway with water and bring it to a boil.

2 Add the mussels and olive oil to the boiling water and continue to boil for 4 minutes. Carefully drain off the water.

3 Pour the dressing over the mussels and serve immediately, garnished with the parsley.

INGREDIENT TIP: As with all live shellfish, pay attention to the telltale opening and closing of shells: Before cooking, they should all be closed, and you should discard any open mussels that don't close up tight when tapped with another mussel. As they cook, the shells will open; be sure to toss out any mussels that haven't opened during the cooking process.

PER SERVING

Macronutrients: Fat 70%; Protein 24%; Carbs 6%
Calories: 230; Total Fat: 18g; Protein: 14g; Total Carbs: 3g; Fiber: 1g; Net Carbs: 2g

THREE-MINUTE LOBSTER TAIL

— SERVES 2 —

I cannot tell you how many people ask me how to cook lobster. And in the same breath, they tell me it's too hard to make. False. It is so easy! Let me show you my method, and you'll be having a seafood feast in no time flat. The trick, as you'll see below, is to cut the lobster shell before cooking. This will allow the lobster to cook without curling and make for easy lobster meat retrieval.

PREP TIME: 5 MINUTES

COOK TIME: 3 MINUTES

– ONE POT

– 30 MINUTES

– 5 INGREDIENTS

4 cups bone broth (or water)

2 lobster tails

1 In a large pot, bring the broth to a boil.

2 While the broth is coming to a boil, use kitchen shears to cut the back side of the lobster shell from end to end.

3 Place the lobster in the boiling broth and bring it back to a boil. Cook the lobster for 3 minutes.

4 Drain and serve immediately.

VARIATION TIP: To serve, plate the whole lobster tail on a bed of lettuce with lemon and radish wedges. Try a drizzle of cacao butter and some freshly ground pepper on top. For a surf-and-turf option, pair with Secret Seasoning Sirloin Steak (page 120) or, as a lighter option, add Prosciutto-Wrapped Asparagus (page 59) and serve Lemon-Garlic Dressing (page 16) on the side, to drizzle over everything.

PER SERVING

Macronutrients: Fat 9%; Protein 89%; Carbs 2%
Calories: 154; Total Fat: 2g; Protein: 32g; Total Carbs: 0g; Fiber: 0g; Net Carbs: 0g

"FRIED" OYSTERS
IN THE OVEN

— SERVES 4 —

Fun fact: I had never had an oyster until I met Brad. Now I eat them every chance I get. Lucky for me, that's fairly often. Even if you're not a fan of raw shellfish, there are plenty of ways to enjoy these treasures, such as this oven-fried method. I like to serve them with Turnip Fries (page 63) and Easiest Tartar Sauce (page 19).

PREP TIME: 20 MINUTES

COOK TIME: 30 MINUTES

– 5 INGREDIENTS

3 tablespoons olive oil

1 teaspoon garlic salt

1 teaspoon freshly ground black pepper

1 teaspoon red pepper flakes

2 cups finely crushed pork rinds

24 shucked oysters

1 Preheat the oven to 400°F.

2 In a small bowl, mix together the olive oil, garlic salt, black pepper, and red pepper flakes.

3 Put the crushed pork rinds in a separate bowl.

4 Dip each oyster first in the oil mixture to coat and then in the pork rinds, turning to coat. Arrange the coated oysters on a baking sheet in a single layer with room in between.

5 Bake in the preheated oven for 30 minutes, or until the pork rind "breading" is browned and crisp. Serve hot.

SIMPLIFY IT! I'm going to be totally honest here: Shucking oysters is hard work and takes a lot of practice to get right. If you've never done it before, do yourself a favor and buy already shucked oysters. Most fish markets sell fresh ones—they're usually found in jars in the case alongside the live oysters. They cost a little more, but they're worth it.

PER SERVING

Macronutrients: Fat 64%; Protein 27%; Carbs 9%

Calories: 230; Total Fat: 17g; Protein: 15g; Total Carbs: 5g; Fiber: 0g; Net Carbs: 5g

TUNA WITH GREENS AND BLUEBERRIES

— SERVES 2 —

It may seem unorthodox, but the combination of seared tuna, fresh salad greens, and ripe blueberries is delicious. Tart lemon, creamy ranch dressing, meaty tuna steaks, and sweet fruit all mingle together for a real taste sensation.

PREP TIME: 10 MINUTES

COOK TIME: 5 MINUTES

- ONE POT
- 30 MINUTES
- 5 INGREDIENTS

¼ cup olive oil

2 (4-ounce) tuna steaks

Salt

Freshly ground black pepper

Juice of 1 lemon

4 cups salad greens

¼ cup low-carb, dairy-free ranch dressing (such as Tessemae's)

20 blueberries

1 In a large skillet, heat the oil over medium-high heat.

2 Season the tuna steaks generously with salt and pepper, and add them to the skillet. Cook for 2 to 2½ minutes on each side to sear the outer edges.

3 Squeeze the lemon over the tuna in the pan and then remove the fish.

4 To serve, arrange the greens on 2 serving plates. Top each plate with one of the tuna steaks, 2 tablespoons of the ranch dressing, and 10 of the blueberries.

INGREDIENT TIP: Tuna is best eaten raw or very rare. When you cook a tuna steak, make sure the pan is very hot before you put the fish in, and cook it just until the fish is browned on the outside but still very rare in the middle.

PER SERVING

Macronutrients: Fat 69%; Protein 26%; Carbs 5%
Calories: 549; Total Fat: 41g; Protein: 38g; Total Carbs: 7g; Fiber: 3g; Net Carbs: 4g

ROASTED SHRIMP

— MAKES 24 SHRIMP —

I love all varieties of shrimp. Battered, fried, roasted, you name it.
I'll eat shrimp any way it's presented (or any way I cook it) and any
day of the week. This recipe roasts them in the oven, topped with
a zesty marinade that cooks down into a delectable sauce.

PREP TIME: 5 MINUTES

COOK TIME: 10 MINUTES

– 30 MINUTES

24 raw shrimp, peeled

5 tablespoons olive oil

2 tablespoons white wine vinegar

Juice of 1 lemon

1 tablespoon minced garlic

1 teaspoon salt

1 teaspoon freshly ground
black pepper

1 teaspoon dried parsley

1 teaspoon dried chives

1 Preheat the oven to 425°F. Line a large rimmed baking sheet with parchment paper.

2 Arrange the shrimp in a single layer on the prepared baking sheet.

3 In a small bowl, whisk together the olive oil, vinegar, lemon juice, garlic, salt, pepper, parsley, and chives. Brush the mixture over the shrimp.

4 Roast the shrimp in the preheated oven for 8 to 10 minutes, or until they turn pink and are cooked through. Serve immediately.

PER SERVING (6 SHRIMP)

Macronutrients: Fat 64%; Protein 34%; Carbs 2%
Calories: 267; Total Fat: 19g; Protein: 23g; Total
Carbs: 1g; Fiber: 0g; Net Carbs: 1g

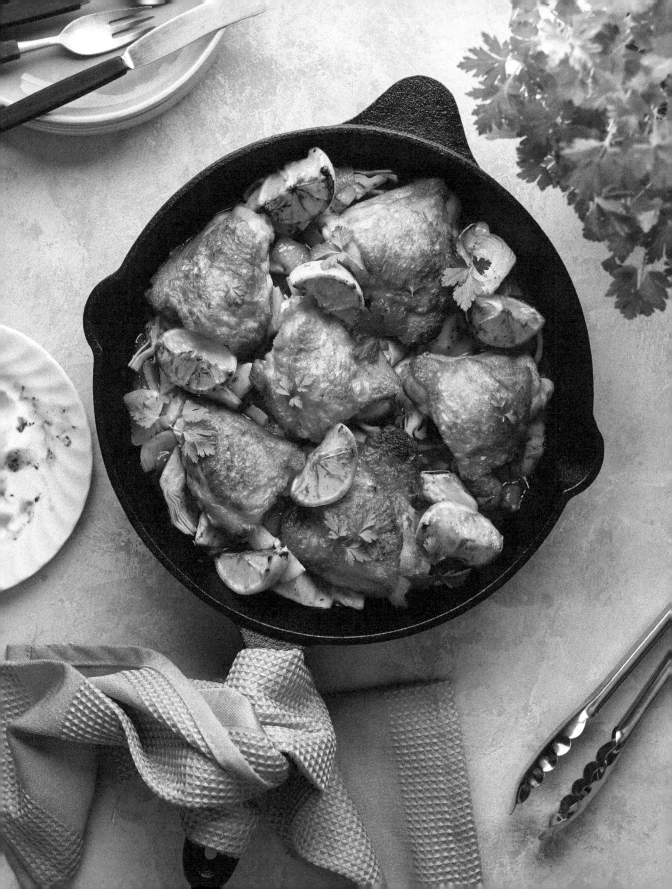

poultry

Opposite: Black Skillet Chicken Thighs with Artichoke Hearts, page 108

SLOW-COOKER BUFFALO CHICKEN

— SERVES 8 —

This is my go-to slow-cooker meal for any occasion, whether it's a party or a low-key night at home. It's always a hit, and super versatile to boot. Eat it on its own with a veggie side and dairy-free ranch dressing, or use it as a dip with sliced bell peppers. You can also scoop the chicken mixture into a hollowed-out green pepper and bake it for 20 minutes at 350°F for a spicy stuffed-pepper dinner.

PREP TIME: 10 MINUTES

COOK TIME: 4 HOURS ON HIGH OR
7 HOURS ON LOW

– ONE POT

– 5 INGREDIENTS

6 boneless, skinless chicken breasts

1 cup hot wing sauce (such as
Frank's RedHot)

1 (8-ounce) containeer dairy-free
cream cheese (such as Kite Hill)

1 onion, diced (optional)

¼ cup olive oil

1 In the slow cooker, combine the chicken, hot sauce, cream cheese, onion (if using), and olive oil. Cover and cook on low for 7 hours or on high for 4 hours.

2 Once cooked, transfer the chicken breasts to a cutting board and use two forks to shred the meat. Return the meat to the sauce in the pot.

3 Serve hot, as a dip, with a side, or straight from the bowl.

PER SERVING

Macronutrients: Fat 58%; Protein 40%; Carbs 2%
Calories: 218; Total Fat: 14g; Protein: 22g; Total
Carbs: 1g; Fiber: 0g; Net Carbs: 1g

SALT-AND-PEPPER CHICKEN KEBABS WITH PINEAPPLE

— SERVES 6 —

I love combining tropical fruit with chicken and vegetables for a fun sweet-savory flavor combo. These kebabs are easy to bake in the oven, or they can be cooked on the grill to give them an added smokiness.

PREP TIME: 15 MINUTES

COOK TIME: 30 MINUTES

– 5 INGREDIENTS

6 boneless, skinless chicken breasts, cut into 2-inch pieces

¼ cup olive oil, plus 2 tablespoons more for greasing the skewers

2 teaspoons salt

1 teaspoon freshly ground black pepper

12 (2-inch) chunks pineapple

1 green bell pepper, seeded and cut into squares

1 onion, cut into 2-inch pieces

8 ounces whole mushrooms

1 Preheat the oven to 400°F.

2 In a large bowl, toss the chicken pieces with the olive oil, salt, and pepper.

3 Grease 6 metal skewers with olive oil (so the chicken will be easier to remove when you eat it later). Thread the pineapple, chicken, pepper, onion, and mushrooms onto the skewers, starting and ending each skewer with pineapple.

4 Lay the skewers on a large rimmed baking sheet and cover with the remaining 2 tablespoons oil. Bake for 30 minutes, or until browned and cooked through.

PER SERVING

Macronutrients: Fat 52%; Protein 38%; Carbs 10%

Calories: 293; Total Fat: 17g; Protein: 28g; Total Carbs: 7g; Fiber: 3g; Net Carbs: 4g

UMAMI CHICKEN BURGERS

— SERVES 4 —

I cannot even begin to tell you how much I love these burgers. The fish sauce is a great addition to the ground chicken, turning what could be a boring recipe into something truly standout. I often triple the recipe and make a dozen or so burgers. They keep in the refrigerator for up to a week, and they're good hot or cold.

PREP TIME: 10 MINUTES

COOK TIME: 20 MINUTES

– 30 MINUTES

– 5 INGREDIENTS

5 tablespoons olive oil, divided

12 ounces spinach

1 pound ground chicken

¼ cup fish sauce (I like Red Boat; see tip)

1 Heat 3 tablespoons of olive oil in a large skillet over medium heat. Add the spinach and sauté until wilted, about 2 minutes. Transfer the spinach to a medium bowl and let cool.

2 Once the spinach has cooled, add the chicken and fish sauce to it, and mix well with your hands. Form the mixture into 4 patties.

3 Heat the remaining 2 tablespoons of olive oil in the skillet over medium heat. Add the meat patties to the skillet and cook for about 4 minutes per side, or until browned and cooked through. Serve immediately or wrap and refrigerate for up to 1 week.

INGREDIENT TIP: Vietnamese fish sauce (*nuoc mam*) is known for its rich umami flavor—it adds that special savory something that makes everything extra delicious. Red Boat Fish Sauce, available at grocery stores, is my favorite.

PER SERVING

Macronutrients: Fat 70%; Protein 25%; Carbs 5%
Calories: 351; Total Fat: 27g; Protein: 23g; Total Carbs: 4g; Fiber: 2g; Net Carbs: 2g

BEST FRIED CHICKEN EVER

— SERVES 4 TO 6 —

When you're craving crispy fried chicken, this recipe has you covered.
Infuse the chicken with flavor by marinating it in pickle juice (genius,
right?), then coat it in almond flour and spices before frying to crispy,
crunchy perfection. Don't be surprised if your friends start jumping on
the keto bandwagon just so they have an excuse to eat this chicken.

PREP TIME: 3 HOURS (OR OVERNIGHT)
COOK TIME: 30 TO 40 MINUTES

8 to 10 boneless, skin-on chicken
thighs or boneless, skinless breasts
(or a combo)

1 cup dill pickle juice

¾ cup almond flour

2 tablespoons minced garlic

2 teaspoons freshly ground
black pepper

2 teaspoons paprika

1½ teaspoons salt

1 teaspoon dry mustard

¾ cup olive oil

1 In a large bowl or plastic bag, combine the
chicken with the pickle juice and refrigerate for
at least 3 hours or, ideally, overnight.

2 In a large bowl, combine the almond flour,
garlic, pepper, paprika, salt, and dry mustard.

3 Heat the oil in a large skillet over medium-
high heat.

4 While the oil is heating, remove the chicken
from the marinade, shaking off any excess and
discarding the marinade. Coat each piece of
chicken in the flour mixture. Add the coated
chicken to the skillet. Reduce the heat to
medium-low and cook the chicken, turning it
every 5 minutes or so, until it's browned and
crispy, about 20 minutes.

5 Transfer the chicken to a paper towel–lined
plate to drain. Serve hot.

VARIATION TIP: Fry up small chunks of
chicken breast to make chicken nuggets. Kids
love these, especially if you serve them with
sugar-free ketchup for dunking.

PER SERVING

Macronutrients: Fat 76%; Protein 20%; Carbs 4%
Calories: 524; Total Fat: 44g; Protein: 26g; Total
Carbs: 6g; Fiber: 3g; Net Carbs: 3g

CHICKEN MEATBALL MARINARA WITH BEAN SPROUTS AND BROCCOLI

— SERVES 6 —

I used to love spaghetti and meatballs with broccoli in my pre-keto days. To adapt it for dairy-free keto, I traded spaghetti for bean sprouts, and I swear it's just as good. It's heartier, too, and made in one pot. Simple is the name of the game, and this is at the top of my list.

PREP TIME: 20 MINUTES

COOK TIME: 45 MINUTES

– ONE POT

– 5 INGREDIENTS

1 pound ground chicken

¼ cup olive oil

2 cups chopped broccoli

1 (24-ounce) jar low-carb marinara sauce (I like Rao's Homemade)

1 (12-ounce) bag bean sprouts (see tip)

1 Form the ground chicken into 12 meatballs.

2 In a large skillet, heat the oil over medium-high heat. Add the meatballs and cook, turning occasionally, until browned, about 8 minutes. Add the broccoli and marinara sauce. Reduce the heat to low, cover, and let simmer for 30 minutes.

3 Add the bean sprouts, increase the heat to medium, and cook, uncovered, for 15 more minutes. Serve hot.

SUBSTITUTION TIP: You can substitute shirataki noodles (such as Miracle Noodles) for the bean sprouts, if you like. Made from the konjac plant, they're low in calories and contain almost no digestible carbohydrates—win-win!

PER SERVING

Macronutrients: Fat 55%; Protein 29%; Carbs 16%
Calories: 247; Total Fat: 15g; Protein: 18g; Total Carbs: 10g; Fiber: 4g; Net Carbs: 6g

GARLIC CHICKEN WINGS

— SERVES 6 —

These oven-baked garlicky wings make great party food, and the recipe
is so simple, you'll soon have it memorized. Cooking the wings from
frozen not only cuts down on prep time but also keeps the meat moist and
tender. Add a dish of dairy-free ranch dressing for dipping, if you like.

PREP TIME: 10 MINUTES

COOK TIME: 1 HOUR

– 5 INGREDIENTS

24 frozen chicken wings

1 cup olive oil

6 garlic cloves, minced

1½ teaspoons salt

1 teaspoon freshly ground
black pepper

1 Preheat the oven to 400°F. Place a baking
rack on top of a large baking sheet.

2 In a large bowl, combine the frozen wings
with the olive oil, garlic, salt, and pepper.

3 Arrange the chicken pieces on top of the
baking rack on the baking sheet. Bake in the
preheated oven for 1 hour, or until browned
and crisp.

PER SERVING

Macronutrients: Fat 78%; Protein 22%; Carbs 0%
Calories: 880; Total Fat: 76g; Protein: 48g; Total
Carbs: 1g; Fiber: 0g; Net Carbs: 1g

BLACK SKILLET CHICKEN THIGHS WITH ARTICHOKE HEARTS

— SERVES 6 —

This is a simple and beautiful one-pot dinner. The trick is to use a black (not enameled) cast iron skillet to brown the chicken to a pretty caramel color on the stovetop, then pop the skillet right into the oven to finish cooking. My cast iron pan was once my grandmother's; I never knew her, but I like to imagine all the meals she cooked with it—though I bet they weren't keto!

PREP TIME: 10 MINUTES

COOK TIME: 50 MINUTES

– ONE POT

– 5 INGREDIENTS

6 tablespoons olive oil

6 boneless, skin-on chicken thighs

1 (14-ounce) can artichoke hearts, drained

1 onion, diced

½ cup bone broth

1 teaspoon salt

1 teaspoon freshly ground black pepper

Juice of 1 lemon

1 Preheat the oven to 400°F.

2 Heat the olive oil in a large cast iron skillet over medium-high heat. Add the chicken and cook until nicely browned on the bottom, about 4 minutes.

3 Once browned, flip the chicken over and add the artichokes, onion, broth, salt, and pepper.

4 Place the skillet in the preheated oven and cook for 40 minutes, or until the chicken is cooked through.

5 Remove the skillet from the oven and squeeze the lemon juice over the top. Serve hot.

VARIATION TIP: Roast a few lemon quarters by adding them to the skillet just before it goes in the oven; serve alongside, with a sprinkling of parsley.

PER SERVING

Macronutrients: Fat 73%; Protein 21%; Carbs 6% Calories: 479; Total Fat: 39g; Protein: 25g; Total Carbs: 7g; Fiber: 4g; Net Carbs: 3g

MOM'S CHICKEN WITH DRIED BEEF AND BACON

— SERVES 12 —

This was a staple entrée when I was growing up. Anytime we had friends over, it was Mom's chicken, mashed potatoes, and green beans. This is my cleaned-up version—I serve it with Cauliflower Mash (page 70) for maximum macro impact—but it still boasts the same flavor and, most importantly, takes me back to that long wooden table and the steam coming off Mom's chicken.

PREP TIME: 20 MINUTES

COOK TIME: 1 HOUR

6 large boneless, skinless chicken breasts, each cut in half

1 (2-ounce) jar or can dried beef

12 strips bacon

1¼ cups bone broth

1 (8-ounce) container dairy-free cream cheese with chives (such as Kite Hill)

1 celery stalk, diced

½ cup canned coconut milk

1 teaspoon freshly ground black pepper

1 Preheat the oven to 375°F.

2 Wrap each piece of chicken with 2 pieces of dried beef, and then with 1 slice of bacon. Arrange the wrapped chicken pieces in a baking dish.

3 In a medium bowl, mix together the broth, cream cheese, celery, coconut milk, and pepper. Pour the mixture over the chicken pieces.

4 Bake, uncovered, in the preheated oven for 1 hour, or until the chicken is cooked through.

INGREDIENT TIP: You can find dried beef in the supermarket, in the same section as the canned tuna. For the coconut milk, if you open a new can for this recipe, use the thick cream that has risen to the top.

PER SERVING

Macronutrients: Fat 62%; Protein 36%; Carbs 2%
Calories: 309; Total Fat: 21g; Protein: 28g; Total Carbs: 2g; Fiber: 0g; Net Carbs: 2g

CHILI-GARLIC CHICKEN WITH BROCCOLI

— SERVES 6 —

Chicken can get boring, but this slow-cooker recipe will remind you how good it can be. It's loaded with veggies and livened up with a spicy sauce. Serve it over cauliflower rice or zucchini noodles. You can find Chinese chili-garlic sauce in the international-foods aisle of most supermarkets.

PREP TIME: 10 MINUTES

COOK TIME: 6 HOURS

− ONE POT

6 boneless, skinless chicken breasts (about 1¼ pounds total), cut into bite-size pieces

1 head broccoli, chopped

8 ounces whole mushrooms

1 large onion, diced

2 cups bone broth

½ cup coconut aminos

5 tablespoons chili-garlic sauce

¼ cup avocado oil

2 tablespoons fish sauce (such as Red Boat)

1 teaspoon minced garlic

½ teaspoon grated fresh ginger

In a slow cooker, combine the chicken, broccoli, mushrooms, onion, bone broth, coconut aminos, chili-garlic sauce, avocado oil, fish sauce, garlic, and ginger. Cover and cook on low for 6 hours. Serve hot.

INGREDIENT TIP: The broccoli in this dish turns out very soft and almost melts into the sauce. If you prefer your broccoli crisp-tender, add it about 30 minutes before the end of the cooking time.

PER SERVING
Macronutrients: Fat 39%; Protein 47%; Carbs 14%
Calories: 244; Total Fat: 11g; Protein: 29g; Total Carbs: 12g; Fiber: 3g; Net Carbs: 9g

POPPY SEED CHICKEN

— SERVES 8 —

Poppy Seed Chicken with a side of green beans might actually be my favorite thing ever. It reminds me of Thanksgiving, even though there's no turkey involved. Something about the rich, creamy sauce makes me feel like my favorite holiday is just around the bend; I can practically hear the clatter of the serving spoons as everyone gathers to pick at the serving platters.

PREP TIME: 20 MINUTES

COOK TIME: 45 MINUTES

2 tablespoons olive oil, plus more for greasing the baking dish

6 boneless, skinless chicken breasts (about 2 pounds), cooked and shredded

1 (8-ounce) container dairy-free cream cheese (such as Kite Hill)

1 cup bone broth

8 ounces mushrooms, sliced

1 14-ounce can coconut milk

2 tablespoons olive oil

1½ teaspoons garlic salt

2 tablespoons poppy seeds

¼ cup slivered almonds

1 Preheat the oven to 350°F. Grease a 9-by-13-inch baking dish.

2 Arrange the shredded chicken in an even layer in the prepared baking dish.

3 In a medium saucepan over low heat, soften the cream cheese, stirring constantly. Once the cheese is melted, stir in the bone broth, mushrooms, coconut milk, olive oil, and garlic salt.

4 Continue cooking on low until the sauce is well combined and thickened. Remove from the heat and stir in the poppy seeds.

5 Immediately pour the sauce over the shredded chicken in the baking dish. Sprinkle the almonds over the top and bake in the preheated oven for 40 minutes, or until bubbly.

PER SERVING

Macronutrients: Fat 63%; Protein 31%; Carbs 6%
Calories: 374; Total Fat: 26g; Protein: 29g; Total Carbs: 7g; Fiber: 1g; Net Carbs: 6g

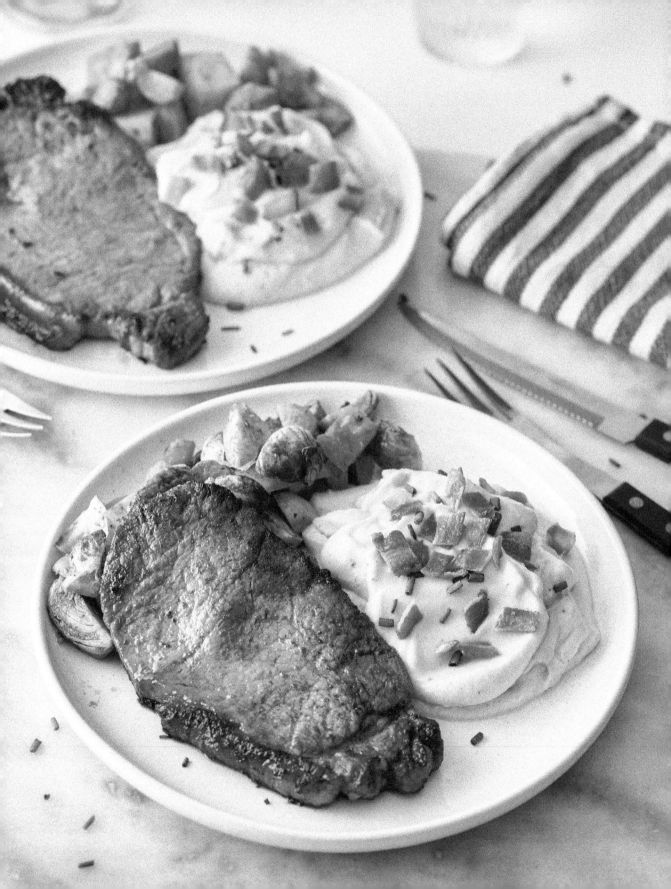

beef

Opposite: Secret Seasoning Sirloin Steak, page 120; Cauliflower Mash, page 70

DINNER ROAST WITH VEGETABLES

— SERVES 8 —

A roast is the ultimate comfort-food dinner, and cooking it in the slow cooker while you're at work might just be the greatest kitchen hack ever invented. Coming home to this kind of dinner is like being welcomed with a kiss at the door from your favorite companion, whether that's your spouse or your puppy.

PREP TIME: 15 MINUTES

COOK TIME: 8 TO 10 HOURS

– ONE POT

1 (3-pound) chuck roast

1 bunch radishes (about 12), diced

2 cups bone broth

5 celery stalks, chopped

8 ounces mushrooms, diced

1 onion, diced

¼ cup coconut aminos

½ cup dairy-free ranch dressing (such as Tessemae's)

1 In a slow cooker, combine the chuck roast, radishes, bone broth, celery, mushrooms, onion, coconut aminos, and ranch dressing.

2 Cover and cook on low for 8 to 10 hours, or until the meat can be easily pulled apart with a fork.

PER SERVING

Macronutrients: Fat 42%; Protein 49%; Carbs 5%
Calories: 383; Total Fat: 18g; Protein: 47g; Total
Carbs: 5g; Fiber 1g; Net Carbs: 4g

TACO SALAD NACHOS

— SERVES 5 —

I've traded in my once-beloved chips and queso, but I'll happily devour this dairy-free keto version of nachos any day. With lots of toppings and the crunch of bell peppers, it makes a great, healthy alternative to salty chips and cheese.

PREP TIME: 10 MINUTES

COOK TIME: 20 MINUTES

– ONE POT

– 30 MINUTES

¼ cup avocado oil

1 pound ground beef

¼ cup dairy-free cream cheese (such as Kite Hill)

1 (14-ounce) can diced tomatoes

1 (12-ounce) bag spinach

1 onion, diced

1 tablespoon minced garlic

1 tablespoon ground cumin

1 teaspoon salt

1 teaspoon freshly ground black pepper

1 red bell pepper, seeded and cut into strips

1 green bell pepper, seeded and cut into strips

1 tablespoon chopped fresh cilantro, for garnish

1 In a large skillet, heat the oil over medium heat. Add the ground beef and cook, stirring, until browned, about 5 minutes. Add the cream cheese and stir until the cheese is melted and creamy.

2 Stir in the tomatoes, spinach, onion, garlic, cumin, salt, and pepper. Cook, stirring frequently, for about 8 minutes more, or until the spinach is wilted and the onion is softened.

3 Arrange the bell peppers on a serving platter. Pour the meat mixture over the peppers and serve hot, garnished with the cilantro.

PER SERVING

Macronutrients: Fat 65%; Protein 25%; Carbs 10%
Calories: 427; Total Fat: 31g; Protein: 27g; Total Carbs: 10g; Fiber: 5g; Net Carbs: 5g

REUBEN WRAPS

— MAKES 12 WRAPS —

If I had to pick a last meal, it would probably be a Reuben sandwich. For this keto-friendly version, I use thick slices of corned beef as the wrap, leave out the cheese, and whip up a dairy-free Thousand Island dressing. The classic combo of sweet relish and tangy sauerkraut really hits the spot.

PREP TIME: 20 MINUTES

COOK TIME: 30 MINUTES

FOR THE DRESSING

1 cup sugar-free mayonnaise (such as Primal Kitchen)

5 tablespoons sugar-free ketchup (such as Primal Kitchen)

¼ cup sweet pickle relish

3 tablespoons white vinegar

2 teaspoons Swerve granular (or other granulated alternative sweetener)

1 teaspoon freshly ground black pepper

FOR THE WRAPS

1 (8-ounce) container dairy-free cream cheese (such as Kite Hill)

2 cups sauerkraut

12 pieces thick-sliced corned beef

TO MAKE THE DRESSING

In a large mixing bowl, stir together the mayonnaise, ketchup, relish, vinegar, sweetener, and pepper.

TO MAKE THE WRAPS

1 Preheat the oven to 350°F.

2 Divide the cream cheese and sauerkraut equally among the 12 slices of corned beef. Add a generous dollop of the dressing.

3 Roll the wraps up and place them in a 9-inch square baking dish, tightly nested together.

4 Cover the baking dish with aluminum foil and cook for 30 minutes, or until the meat is crispy on the edges.

INGREDIENT TIP: Be generous with the dressing in these wraps! Don't worry, you can't overfill these babies.

PER SERVING (3 WRAPS)

Macronutrients: Fat 68%; Protein 17%; Carbs 15%

Calories: 372; Total Fat: 28g; Protein: 16g;

Total Carbs: 14g; Fiber: 4g; Net Carbs: 10g;

Erythritol 0.5g

CLASSIC KETO MEAT LOAF

— SERVES 6 —

This meat loaf makes a great dinner, but it also makes perfect leftovers. I usually serve it with a side of Cauliflower Mash (page 70) the first night and then eat it in lettuce wraps with sugar-free ketchup for lunch the next day.

PREP TIME: 10 MINUTES

COOK TIME: 1 HOUR

Oil, for greasing the baking sheet

1 pound ground beef

½ onion, diced

½ green bell pepper, seeded and diced

⅔ cup sugar-free ketchup (such as Primal Kitchen), divided

1 large egg

1 teaspoon dried sage

1 teaspoon dry mustard

1 teaspoon salt

1 teaspoon freshly ground black pepper

1 Preheat the oven to 350°F. Grease a large rimmed baking sheet.

2 In a large bowl, mix together the ground beef, onion, green pepper, ⅓ cup of ketchup, the egg, sage, dry mustard, salt, and pepper. Form the mixture into a loaf on the baking sheet, and then top it with the remaining ⅓ cup of ketchup.

3 Cook in the preheated oven for 1 hour. Let rest for 5 to 10 minutes before slicing.

SUBSTITUTION TIP: You can substitute another ground meat for the beef, such as ground turkey or pork, or you can use a combination. I like to mix beef and lamb.

PER SERVING

Macronutrients: Fat 72%; Protein 22%; Carbs 6% Calories: 260; Total Fat: 21g; Protein: 13g; Total Carbs: 4g; Fiber: 1g; Net Carbs: 3g

BEEF LIVER BURGERS

— SERVES 4 TO 6 —

Don't be intimidated by beef liver—it's a nutrition powerhouse and packs tons of flavor. Adding it to your burgers not only makes them superrich and tasty but also adds B vitamins (including B_{12}), protein, zinc, copper, iron, and even vitamin C. These nourishing burgers are meaty and finger-licking good—exactly what burgers should be.

PREP TIME: 10 MINUTES

COOK TIME: 20 MINUTES

– 30 MINUTES

– 5 INGREDIENTS

1 pound ground beef or bison

8 ounces beef liver, cut into small pieces

3 tablespoons sugar-free ketchup (such as Primal Kitchen)

3 teaspoons garlic salt, divided

3 tablespoons olive oil

1 In a small bowl, combine the ground meat, liver, ketchup, and 2 teaspoons of garlic salt. Mix well and form into 4 to 6 burger patties.

2 In a cast iron skillet, heat the oil over medium heat. Add the burgers, then sprinkle them with the remaining teaspoon of garlic salt. Cook for 8 to 10 minutes per side, or until cooked through. Serve hot.

VARIATION TIP: Top each burger with a Homestyle Fried Egg (page 32) and serve it with all your favorite sugar-free burger fixings.

PER SERVING

Macronutrients: Fat 74%; Protein 24%; Carbs 2%
Calories: 497; Total Fat: 41g; Protein: 30g; Total Carbs: 2g; Fiber: 0g; Net Carbs: 2g

PHILLY CHEESESTEAK BAKE

— SERVES 8 —

Everyone loves a Philly cheesesteak, so, of course, I had to make a dairy-free keto version. It's further proof that just about any dish can be adapted for this way of eating. Believe it or not, it's amazing and even easy. If you don't tell people it's dairy-free, they'll never know.

PREP TIME: 10 MINUTES

COOK TIME: 30 MINUTES

2 tablespoons olive oil, plus more for greasing the baking dish

1 (8-ounce) container dairy-free cream cheese (such as Kite Hill)

¾ cup sugar-free mayonnaise (such as Primal Kitchen)

¼ cup canned coconut milk or nut milk

¼ cup whole-grain mustard

2 tablespoons minced garlic

2 tablespoons olive oil

1 tomato, chopped

1 green bell pepper, seeded and chopped

1 onion, diced

8 ounces mushrooms, chopped

1½ pounds deli-sliced roast beef, chopped

1 Preheat the oven to 400°F. Grease a 9-by-13-inch baking dish.

2 In a medium bowl, stir together the cream cheese, mayonnaise, coconut milk, mustard, and garlic until well combined.

3 Heat the olive oil in a large skillet over medium heat. Add the tomato, green pepper, onion, and mushrooms. Cook, stirring frequently, until the vegetables are softened, about 8 minutes.

4 Spread the roast beef in an even layer in the prepared baking dish. Top with the vegetable mixture and then the cream cheese mixture. Bake in the preheated oven for 20 minutes, or until the dish is hot and bubbly.

PER SERVING

Macronutrients: Fat 71%; Protein 25%; Carbs 4%
Calories: 534; Total Fat: 42g; Protein: 34g; Total Carbs: 5g; Fiber: 2g; Net Carbs: 3g

SECRET SEASONING SIRLOIN STEAK

— SERVES 2 —

My dad always put ketchup and garlic salt on steaks to season them, and I fondly remember how every time we had company, our guests would go on and on about his steak's secret seasonings. My dad was a humble man, but, funnily enough, I never heard him say, "Oh, it's just ketchup!" I think he wanted it to be his secret. Sorry, Dad—some secrets just can't be kept forever.

PREP TIME: 5 MINUTES

COOK TIME: 20 MINUTES

– 30 MINUTES

– 5 INGREDIENTS

2 (6- to 8-ounce) sirloin steaks, at room temperature

¼ cup sugar-free ketchup (such as Primal Kitchen)

4 teaspoons garlic salt

¼ cup olive oil

1 Heat the broiler to high.

2 Lay out the steaks on a plate and cover each side with the ketchup and garlic salt.

3 In a cast iron skillet, heat the oil over high heat. Add the steaks and cook for 1 minute on each side.

4 Transfer the skillet to the broiler and cook for 5 minutes more.

5 Remove the skillet from the oven, flip the steaks over, and let them continue to cook in the hot pan for 10 more minutes.

6 Serve immediately.

SIMPLIFY IT! Use a splatter screen (see page 8) so the grease won't splash—it'll keep cleanup easy, too.

PER SERVING

Macronutrients: Fat 67%; Protein 31%; Carbs 2%
Calories: 462; Total Fat: 34g; Protein: 36g; Total Carbs: 3g; Fiber: 0g; Net Carbs: 3g

SLOPPY JOES

— SERVES 4 —

One day, my husband was craving sloppy joes, which had never been a favorite of mine. Because I like to be nice to him, I whipped up this keto version— only to be surprised by how much I loved it. I leave out the bun altogether, but I do like to serve it with Turnip Fries (page 63) to complete the dish.

PREP TIME: 10 MINUTES

COOK TIME: 30 MINUTES

– ONE POT

1 pound ground beef

1 onion, diced

¾ cup sugar-free ketchup (such as Primal Kitchen)

2 tablespoons garlic powder

1 tablespoon white vinegar

1 tablespoon Swerve granular (or other granulated alternative sweetener)

1 Heat a large skillet over medium-high heat. Add the meat and cook, stirring, until it begins to brown, about 3 minutes. Add the onion and cook, stirring frequently, until the meat is browned and the onion is softened, about 5 minutes.

2 Stir in the ketchup, garlic powder, vinegar, and sweetener. Reduce the heat to medium-low and cook for 20 minutes more. Serve hot.

VARIATION TIP: If you want a true sloppy joe experience, serve this on top of toasted slices of low-carb bread.

PER SERVING

Macronutrients: Fat 75%; Protein 21%; Carbs 4% Calories: 356; Total Fat: 28g; Protein: 19g; Total Carbs: 4g; Fiber: 1g; Net Carbs: 3g; Erythritol 3g

CABBAGE SLAW WITH GROUND BEEF

— SERVES 4 —

This meaty cabbage slaw is great served hot or cold, so it's another one that's ideal for making in a large batch and enjoying as leftovers all week. The fish sauce lends extra umami richness to the dish.

PREP TIME: 5 MINUTES

COOK TIME: 30 MINUTES

– ONE POT

– 5 INGREDIENTS

3 tablespoons olive oil

1 pound ground beef

1 (16-ounce) bag cabbage slaw mix

3 tablespoons coconut aminos

1 tablespoon fish sauce (such as Red Boat)

1 Heat the olive oil in a large skillet over medium-high heat. Add the meat and cook, stirring, until browned, about 7 minutes. Add the cabbage and cook, stirring occasionally, until wilted, about 15 minutes.

2 Stir in the coconut aminos and fish sauce, and simmer for 5 minutes more.

3 Serve hot or cover and store in the refrigerator for up to 5 days.

PER SERVING

Macronutrients: Fat 76%; Protein 16%; Carbs 8%
Calories: 463; Total Fat: 39g; Protein: 18g; Total Carbs: 10g; Fiber: 4g; Net Carbs: 6g

CHEESEBURGER HASH

— SERVES 10 —

Cheeseburger Hash is a guilty pleasure, and I refuse to live my life without it. I created this dairy-free keto version so that I wouldn't have to, and now it appears almost weekly at our dinner table. Naturally, Turnip Fries (page 63) make the perfect side.

PREP TIME: 20 MINUTES

COOK TIME: 50 MINUTES

3 tablespoons olive oil, plus more for greasing the baking dish

2 pounds ground beef

1 (16-ounce) bag cabbage slaw mix

1 large onion, diced

8 ounces mushrooms, sliced

1 (8-ounce) container dairy-free cream cheese with chives (such as Kite Hill)

1 cup canned coconut milk

3 tablespoons nutritional yeast

2 teaspoons granulated garlic

1 teaspoon salt

1 teaspoon freshly ground black pepper

1 batch Perfect Bacon (page 31), crumbled

1 Preheat the oven to 350°F. Grease a 9-by-13-inch baking dish.

2 Heat the oil in a large skillet over medium-high heat. Add the meat, cabbage slaw mix, onion, and mushrooms, and cook, stirring frequently, for 15 to 20 minutes, or until the meat is browned and the vegetables are softened.

3 Transfer the mixture to the prepared baking dish.

4 In a large microwave-safe bowl, heat the cream cheese for 40 seconds in the microwave to soften.

5 To the bowl with the cream cheese, add the coconut milk, nutritional yeast, garlic, salt, and pepper, and whisk to combine well.

6 Pour the cream cheese mixture over the meat and vegetables in the baking dish. Bake in the preheated oven for 30 minutes, or until bubbling and lightly browned on top.

7 Serve hot, topped with the bacon.

VARIATION TIP: Serve with anything that might usually top a cheeseburger: sugar-free ketchup, mustard, low-carb mayonnaise, shredded lettuce, sliced tomatoes, and sliced onions.

PER SERVING

Macronutrients: Fat 73%; Protein 21%; Carbs 6%

Calories: 557; Total Fat: 45g; Protein: 29g; Total Carbs: 9g; Fiber: 4g; Net Carbs: 5g

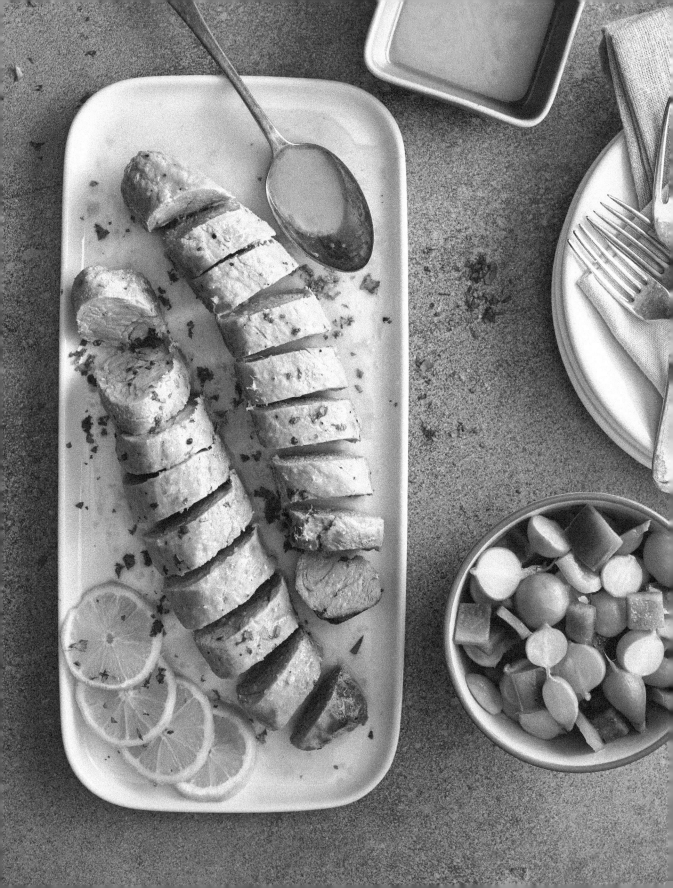

pork

Opposite: Lemon-Garlic Pork Tenderloin with Radishes and Green Pepper, page 129

KIELBASA AND SAUERKRAUT

— SERVES 4 —

This is another dish that always reminds me of my mama and home.
Mom always served this with mashed potatoes, so obviously I love
to pair it with Cauliflower Mash (page 70). It's a simple meal to put
together, and it's also filling—for the belly and the soul.

PREP TIME: 5 MINUTES

COOK TIME: 10 MINUTES

− ONE POT

− 30 MINUTES

− 5 INGREDIENTS

1 (16-ounce) jar or can sauerkraut

1 pound pork kielbasa, diced

2 tablespoons olive oil

In a medium saucepan, bring the sauerkraut to
a boil over medium-high heat. Add the diced
sausage and the olive oil, and simmer over low
heat until heated through, about 5 minutes.

INGREDIENT TIP: If you don't have kielbasa,
you can substitute another type of smoked
sausage—just be sure to check the ingredients
for hidden dairy, sugar, or fillers.

PER SERVING

Macronutrients: Fat 81%; Protein 14%; Carbs 5%
Calories: 435; Total Fat: 39g; Protein: 15g; Total
Carbs: 6g; Fiber: 3g; Net Carbs: 3g

POTLUCK BBQ PORK

— SERVES 7 —

Being from the South, I was born and raised to love good Southern barbecue.
This barbecue pork comes together easily, and it's a great dish to bring
to the next cookout—if you don't decide to keep it all for yourself.

PREP TIME: 10 MINUTES

COOK TIME: 8 HOURS

– ONE POT

1 (2-pound) whole pork shoulder

2 (6-ounce) cans tomato paste

1 white onion, diced

1 cup low-carb tomato sauce

1 batch Red Pepper Dry Rub (page 14)

3 tablespoons white vinegar

2 tablespoons coconut aminos

2 tablespoons whole-grain mustard

1 In a large slow cooker, combine the pork, tomato paste, onion, tomato sauce, dry rub, vinegar, coconut aminos, and mustard.

2 Cover and cook on low for 8 hours.

3 Once cooked, remove the meat and shred it using a hand mixer or two forks. Return the meat to the pot and stir to mix well. Serve hot.

SIMPLIFY IT! If you want an even easier recipe, skip most of the ingredients. Just use the pork shoulder and 2 (10-ounce) bottles of Tessemae's barbecue sauce or your favorite low-carb sauce.

PER SERVING
Macronutrients: Fat 60%; Protein 32%; Carbs 8%
Calories: 342; Total Fat: 22g; Protein: 26g; Total
Carbs: 10g; Fiber: 4g; Net Carbs: 6g

GARLIC PORK CHOPS WITH ONION-AND-MUSHROOM GRAVY

— SERVES 4 —

My mom used to make pork chops and creamy gravy for Sunday dinner, so it's another dish that always reminds me of my childhood. I use coconut milk here to thicken the gravy and get that delectable richness without adding any dairy.

PREP TIME: 10 MINUTES
COOK TIME: 1 HOUR

¼ cup garlic powder

1 teaspoon salt

1 teaspoon freshly ground black pepper

½ teaspoon cayenne

4 pork chops

¼ cup olive oil

8 ounces whole mushrooms

1 onion, diced

2 cups bone broth

¼ cup coconut milk

1 In a small bowl, mix together the garlic powder, salt, pepper, and cayenne.

2 Coat the pork chops with the spice rub mixture, using all of the mixture.

3 Heat the oil in a large cast iron skillet over medium heat. Add the mushrooms and onion and cook, stirring frequently, until softened, about 8 minutes. Add the broth and cook for 20 minutes, or until the liquid is reduced by about half.

4 Increase the heat to high and add the pork chops. Cook for 8 to 10 minutes on each side, depending on the thickness of the pork chop, or until browned and cooked through.

5 Remove the chops from the skillet, but continue to cook the vegetables in the skillet. Add the coconut milk and cook, stirring frequently, for 2 minutes more, or until heated through and combined.

6 Serve the chops with the vegetables and gravy poured over the top.

PER SERVING

Macronutrients: Fat 53%; Protein 38%; Carbs 9%

Calories: 416; Total Fat: 24g; Protein: 40g; Total Carbs: 10g; Fiber: 2g; Net Carbs: 8g

LEMON-GARLIC PORK TENDERLOIN WITH RADISHES AND GREEN PEPPER

— SERVES 8 —

Cooking pork tenderloin all day in a slow cooker with Lemon-Garlic Dressing (page 16) yields tender marinated meat that's great with everything. And coming home to a house full of that delicious aroma is such a treat. This is another dish that makes excellent leftovers for wraps and quick lunches.

PREP TIME: 10 MINUTES

COOK TIME: 8 HOURS

– ONE POT

1 pound pork tenderloin

¼ cup olive oil

1 bunch of radishes (about 12), diced

1 green bell pepper, seeded and diced

1 cup bone broth

¾ cup Lemon-Garlic Dressing (page 16)

4 lemon slices

1 Place the pork in a slow cooker and pour the olive oil over the top. Add the radishes and green bell pepper. Pour the broth and dressing over the top. Lay the lemon slices on top of the pork.

2 Cover and cook on low for 8 hours, or until the pork is very tender.

PER SERVING

Macronutrients: Fat 76%; Protein 21%; Carbs 3%
Calories: 249; Total Fat: 21g; Protein: 13g; Total Carbs: 2g; Fiber: 0g; Net Carbs: 2g

DRY RUB RIBS

— SERVES 6 —

When I created this recipe, I was both pleased and a little bummed. Pleased because it was a huge success—but bummed because now we have no excuse to go get ribs at our favorite barbecue place. Either way, cooking up a full rack of ribs in your kitchen is really good for your culinary self-esteem—and the slow cooker makes this recipe easy-peasy!

PREP TIME: 10 MINUTES

COOK TIME: 8 HOURS

– ONE POT

– 5 INGREDIENTS

1 full rack baby back ribs, cut in half to fit in the pot

6 tablespoons olive oil

2 batches Red Pepper Dry Rub (page 14)

½ cup water

1 Coat the ribs with the oil and then with the dry rub, and put them in a slow cooker with the water.

2 Cover and cook on low for 8 hours. Serve hot.

VARIATION TIP: If you like your ribs wet, serve a dish of dairy-free ranch dressing (such as Tessemae's) on the side for dipping.

PER SERVING

Macronutrients: Fat 86%; Protein 14%; Carbs 0%
Calories: 336; Total Fat: 32g; Protein: 12g; Total Carbs: 0g; Fiber: 0g; Net Carbs: 0g

BACON-WRAPPED "FRIED" PICKLES

— SERVES 12 —

Just when you thought we couldn't go any further down the "I love pickles" rabbit hole, we find ourselves here once again. These are like fried pickles but even better, if you can imagine that, because they're wrapped in savory strips of bacon that crisp up in the oven.

PREP TIME: 5 MINUTES

COOK TIME: 25 MINUTES

- ONE POT

- 30 MINUTES

- 5 INGREDIENTS

12 dill pickle spears

12 strips bacon

1 Preheat the oven to 400°F.

2 Wrap each pickle spear tightly with 1 piece of bacon.

3 Arrange the wrapped pickles on the baking sheet and bake for 25 minutes, or until the bacon is crispy.

4 Place on a wire rack to cool; the pickle juice and bacon fat make for a very hot combination.

PER SERVING

Macronutrients: Fat 71%; Protein 28%; Carbs 1%
Calories: 104; Total Fat: 8g; Protein: 7g; Total Carbs: 1g; Fiber: 0g; Net Carbs: 1g

STUFFED POBLANO PEPPERS

— SERVES 5 —

Poblano peppers are longer and fatter than bell peppers, but almost as mild. They have a great chile flavor without being too spicy. They're easy to work with, and I love them stuffed with ground meat and baked. Here, the pork gets a dash of spice and tomato before going into the peppers.

PREP TIME: 10 MINUTES

COOK TIME: 40 MINUTES

2 tablespoons olive oil, plus more for greasing the baking dish

1 pound ground pork

1 (4-ounce) can diced green chiles

½ cup tomato sauce

1 jalapeño pepper, chopped

1 tablespoon minced garlic

1 teaspoon dried basil

1 teaspoon salt

1 teaspoon freshly ground black pepper

5 poblano peppers

1 Preheat the oven to 400°F. Grease a 9-inch square baking dish.

2 In a large skillet, heat the olive oil over medium-high heat. Add the pork and begin to brown.

3 As the meat begins to brown, add the diced green chiles, tomato sauce, jalapeño, garlic, basil, salt, and pepper. Cook, stirring frequently, until the meat is browned, about 5 minutes.

4 Stuff each poblano pepper with the meat mixture, and arrange the stuffed peppers in the prepared baking dish. Bake in the preheated oven for 30 minutes, or until bubbling and browned on the top.

INGREDIENT TIP: I love spice, so I use a whole jalapeño pepper (seeds and all)—even sometimes 2 or 3! If you like your food milder, take out the ribs and seeds of the jalapeño before chopping.

PER SERVING

Macronutrients: Fat 64%; Protein 26%; Carbs 10%
Calories: 271; Total Fat: 19g; Protein: 18g; Total Carbs: 7g; Fiber: 2g; Net Carbs: 5g

SHEPHERD'S PIE

— SERVES 10 —

Shepherd's Pie is another homey dish that I love to make. On a blustery winter day, it's like a warm hug from a long-lost friend. This keto-friendly version uses Cauliflower Mash (page 70) to replace the traditional mashed potato topping, and it's every bit as good.

PREP TIME: 45 MINUTES

COOK TIME: 8 HOURS

– ONE POT

2 pounds ground sausage

1 (12-ounce) bag spinach

1 cup sliced mushrooms

1 onion, diced

1 cup bone broth

¼ cup coconut aminos

2 tablespoons minced garlic

1 recipe Cauliflower Mash (page 70), prepared but uncooked

1 In a slow cooker, combine the sausage, spinach, mushrooms, onion, broth, coconut aminos, and garlic.

2 Cover and cook on low for 7 hours.

3 Spread the Cauliflower Mash over the meat mixture. Cover and cook for an additional 30 minutes to 1 hour.

4 Serve hot.

PER SERVING

Macronutrients: Fat 76%; Protein 19%; Carbs 5%
Calories: 476; Total Fat: 40g; Protein: 23g; Total Carbs: 6g; Fiber: 2g; Net Carbs: 4g

GROUND-PORK SKILLET WITH ZUCCHINI AND ONION

— SERVES 6 —

Zucchini cook up quickly, and they're super versatile. They add some green and a little more substance to a ground-meat skillet dish, even acting a bit like noodles. For this recipe, I throw them on at the very end to steam just slightly on the finished dish. You can substitute another summer squash if you like.

PREP TIME: 10 MINUTES

COOK TIME: 20 MINUTES

– ONE POT

– 30 MINUTES

– 5 INGREDIENTS

2 tablespoons olive oil

1 pound ground pork

1 large onion, diced

1 cup coconut milk

2 tablespoons minced garlic

1 teaspoon salt

1 teaspoon freshly ground black pepper

15 medium zucchini, spiralized

1 Heat the olive oil in a large skillet over medium-high heat. Add the pork and cook, stirring, until browned, about 5 minutes. Add the onion and cook, stirring frequently, until softened, about 5 more minutes.

2 Stir in the coconut milk, garlic, salt, and pepper. Reduce the heat to low and cook for about 10 more minutes, or until the sauce thickens.

3 Add the zucchini, toss to mix, and serve immediately.

PER SERVING

Macronutrients: Fat 77%; Protein 18%; Carbs 5%
Calories: 329; Total Fat: 29g; Protein: 15g; Total
Carbs: 5g; Fiber: 1g; Net Carbs: 4g

HOLIDAY SAUSAGE BALLS

— MAKES 12 TO 15 BALLS —

These spicy sausage balls are a Christmas favorite at our house. After all, the holidays offer the perfect excuse to eat too many of them. This twist on a traditional sausage ball uses breakfast sausage and lots of spice.

PREP TIME: 15 MINUTES

COOK TIME: 25 MINUTES

– 5 INGREDIENTS

Oil, for greasing the baking sheet

1 pound loose breakfast sausage

2 tablespoons almond flour

1 tablespoon hot wing sauce (such as Frank's RedHot)

1 teaspoon cayenne

1 Preheat the oven to 350ºF. Grease a large rimmed baking sheet.

2 In a medium bowl, thoroughly mix the breakfast sausage, almond flour, hot sauce, and cayenne. Form into bite-size balls and place on the greased baking sheet.

3 Bake for 25 minutes, or until browned and cooked through.

PER SERVING (3 BALLS)
Macronutrients: Fat 78%; Protein 22%; Carbs 0%
Calories: 258; Total Fat: 22g; Protein: 15g; Total Carbs: 0g; Fiber: 0g; Net Carbs: 0g

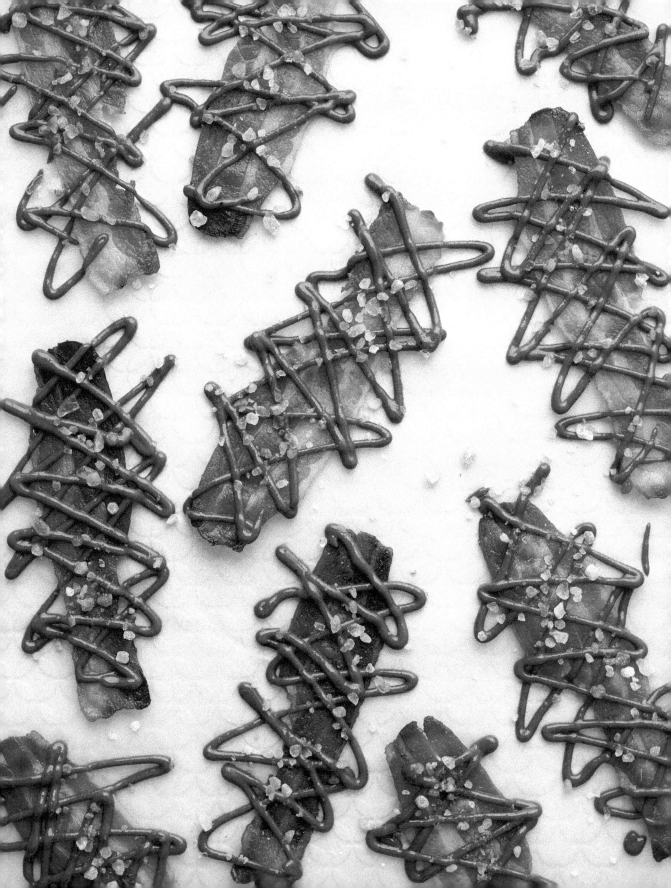

CHAPTER 11

desserts

Opposite: Chocolate Bacon with Pink Himalayan Salt, page 148

GOOD-AS-YOUR-MAMA'S BERRY COBBLER

— SERVES 6 —

I love a good cobbler with ice cream. Unfortunately, a good cobbler with ice cream isn't dairy-free or keto friendly. Enter this recipe, which swaps in coconut milk, cacao butter, and almond flour. (Always remember to eat berries in moderation only.)

PREP TIME: 10 MINUTES

COOK TIME: 30 MINUTES

FOR THE FILLING

1 pint blueberries

½ pint blackberries

¼ cup Swerve granular (or other granulated alternative sweetener)

¼ cup coconut milk

FOR THE CRUST

½ cup cacao butter or coconut oil

¾ cup Swerve granular (or other granulated alternative sweetener), divided

1 large egg

1 teaspoon vanilla extract

½ cup almond flour

1 teaspoon salt

1 teaspoon baking powder

TO MAKE THE FILLING

Toss the blueberries, blackberries, sweetener, and coconut milk together in a 9-inch square baking dish.

TO MAKE THE CRUST

1 In a microwave-safe bowl, melt the cacao butter until liquefied, about 2 minutes. Add ¼ cup of sweetener, the egg, and vanilla, and whisk together until blended well.

2 In another small bowl, combine the remaining ½ cup of sweetener with the almond flour, salt, and baking powder. Add the dry ingredients to the egg mixture and mix to combine.

3 Dollop spoonfuls of the crust mixture over the berry mixture.

4 Bake in the preheated oven for 30 minutes, or until browned on top. Serve hot.

PER SERVING

Macronutrients: Fat 81%; Protein 4%; Carbs 15%
Calories: 241; Total Fat: 22g; Protein: 2g;
Total Carbs: 10g; Fiber: 3g; Net Carbs: 7g;
Erythritol 32g

NO-BAKE HAYSTACK COOKIES

— MAKES 15 TO 18 COOKIES —

My dad used to love the coconut-flake candies he called "haystacks." I was thinking of him when I invented these melt-in-your-mouth coconut cookie wonders. You can keep them in the refrigerator or freezer—I usually opt for the fridge, but there's something fun about a frozen treat, too, especially in the heat of summer.

PREP TIME: 10 MINUTES (PLUS 3 HOURS FOR CHILLING)

– NO COOK

1 (8-ounce) container dairy-free cream cheese (such as Kite Hill)

¾ cup unsweetened shredded coconut

½ cup Swerve granular (or other granulated alternative sweetener)

¼ cup peanut butter

1 tablespoon cacao powder

1 tablespoon chia seeds

1 In a small microwave-safe bowl, melt the cream cheese in the microwave for 30 seconds. Whisk in the coconut, sweetener, peanut butter, cacao powder, and chia seeds.

2 On a baking sheet or plate, form the mixture into small domes, or "haystacks." Chill in the refrigerator for 3 hours (or until you've eaten them all).

PER SERVING (1 COOKIE)

Macronutrients: Fat 84%; Protein 5%; Carbs 11%

Calories: 172; Total Fat: 16g; Protein: 2g; Total Carbs: 5g; Fiber: 3g; Net Carbs: 2g; Erythritol 6g

MACADAMIA NUT BUTTER CUPS

— MAKES 12 CUPS —

I first made these on a whim many years ago, but I have since become a pro because Brad requests them often. I'm happy to oblige, since it means I get to be the taste tester. Macadamia Nut Butter (page 21) is incredibly creamy and buttery; combine it with Chocolate Sauce (page 23) and freeze it, and you'd never guess these tasty morsels are dairy-free.

PREP TIME: 10 MINUTES (PLUS 4 HOURS FOR CHILLING)

– NO COOK

– 5 INGREDIENTS

Coconut oil, for greasing the pan

1 batch Macadamia Nut Butter (page 21)

½ batch Chocolate Sauce (page 23)

1 Grease a silicone muffin pan with coconut oil.

2 Pour the nut butter into the cups, dividing equally. Dampen your hands with cold water and use your fingertips to pat down and flatten the nut butter.

3 Freeze for at least 2 hours, or until hardened.

4 Pour the chocolate sauce over the chilled cups and freeze for at least another 2 hours, or until hardened. Serve straight from the freezer.

VARIATION TIP: Add a tiny sliver of bacon to the top, or some Himalayan salt for a gourmet chocolate-shop twist.

PER SERVING (1 CUP)
Macronutrients: Fat 90%; Protein 4%; Carbs 6%
Calories: 329; Total Fat: 33g; Protein: 3g; Total Carbs: 5g; Fiber: 1g; Net Carbs: 4g

PEANUT BUTTER COOKIES

— MAKES ABOUT 15 COOKIES —

I love the crumbly, nutty sweetness of peanut butter cookies, and
these dairy-free keto ones don't disappoint. For extra indulgence,
you can add a dollop of dark chocolate when you pull them out of the
oven—but I prefer the classic plain cookie, fork print and all.

PREP TIME: 15 MINUTES

COOK TIME: 12 MINUTES

– 30 MINUTES

– 5 INGREDIENTS

¾ cup peanut butter

1 cup Swerve confectioners' (or other
powdered alternative sweetener)

¼ cup olive oil

1 large egg

1 Preheat the oven to 325°F. Line a large baking sheet with parchment paper.

2 In a medium bowl, combine the peanut butter, sweetener, oil, and egg. Mix well.

3 Roll the batter into 1-inch balls and arrange
them on the prepared baking sheet 2 inches
apart. Press the tines of a fork into each cookie
to get the traditional crosshatch design.

4 Bake for 12 minutes, or until lightly browned
and crisp.

VARIATION TIP: Add a sprinkle of Swerve
granular or a few dark chocolate chips while the
cookies are still hot.

PER SERVING (1 COOKIE)
Macronutrients: Fat 76%; Protein 14%; Carbs 10%
Calories: 118; Total Fat: 10g; Protein: 4g; Total
Carbs: 3g; Fiber: 1g; Net Carbs: 2g; Erythritol 13g

PEANUT BUTTER CHOCOLATE PIE

— SERVES 10 —

Peanut butter and chocolate is one of my all-time favorite combinations. This pie combines them beautifully, while still keeping the dish dairy-free and low-carb. This recipe always makes me think of my mother-in-law; it's her favorite pie, and has become a required dessert on our holiday table. Keep it in the freezer through the main course—I like to set it out to thaw about 20 minutes before serving dessert. That way the chocolate makes a hard shell, and it is divine!

PREP TIME: 30 MINUTES

COOK TIME: 15 MINUTES (PLUS 3 HOURS FOR CHILLING)

FOR THE CRUST

3 tablespoons coconut oil, plus more for greasing the pan

1½ cups almonds

1 large egg

FOR THE FILLING

8 ounces peanut butter

8 ounces dairy-free whipped topping

1 (8-ounce) container dairy-free cream cheese (such as Kite Hill)

½ cup Swerve granular (or other granulated alternative sweetener)

FOR THE TOPPING

1 cup cacao butter

2 tablespoons Swerve confectioners' (or other powdered alternative sweetener)

1 heaping tablespoon cacao powder

TO MAKE THE CRUST

1 Preheat the oven to 400°F. Grease a 9-inch pie plate with coconut oil.

2 In a blender or food processor, process the almonds, egg, and oil together until they reach a coarse meal consistency.

3 Press the mixture into the prepared pie plate. Wet your hands with cold water and pat the crust mixture down to cover the dish as evenly as you can.

4 Bake in the preheated oven for 12 minutes. Remove from the oven and let cool.

TO MAKE THE FILLING

1 While baking the crust, in a large mixing bowl, combine the peanut butter, whipped topping, cream cheese, and sweetener and beat until smooth.

2 Pour the mixture into the cooled piecrust. Put in the freezer to chill for at least 1 hour.

TO MAKE THE TOPPING

1 In a small pan over medium-high heat, mix the cacao butter, sweetener, and cacao powder until melted.

2 Pull the pie out of the freezer and pour the chocolate mixture over it.

3 Put the pie back in the freezer and freeze for at least 2 hours. Serve chilled.

VARIATION TIP: You can omit the chocolate if you're not a chocolate person; simply top with a handful of crushed peanuts for a sweet and delectable Peanut Butter Pie. Or keep the chocolate and add a little salty goodness by sprinkling about 1 teaspoon of Himalayan pink salt on top—now it's a Salted Chocolate Peanut Butter Pie, sure to satisfy every craving.

PER SERVING

Macronutrients: Fat 85%; Protein 9%; Carbs 6%
Calories: 557; Total Fat: 53g; Protein: 12g; Total Carbs: 8g; Fiber: 3g; Net Carbs: 5g; Erythritol: 12g

BEST BROWNIES

— MAKES 12 BROWNIES —

I have long been trying to develop a keto-friendly brownie recipe that uses only pantry ingredients—because, let's be honest, when the chocolate urge hits, you need a brownie, stat. These are going to be your new go-to emergency chocolate dessert; they've definitely become mine. No grocery run necessary.

PREP TIME: 10 MINUTES

COOK TIME: 25 MINUTES

1¼ cups Swerve granular (or other granulated alternative sweetener)

½ cup almond flour

½ cup coconut flour

½ cup cacao powder

1 teaspoon baking powder

1 cup olive oil

½ cup plus 2 tablespoons canned coconut milk (shake the can well before opening)

1 large egg

2 teaspoons vanilla extract

1 Preheat the oven to 350°F.

2 In a stand mixer, combine the sweetener, almond flour, coconut flour, cacao powder, and baking powder. With the mixer running, add the olive oil, coconut milk, egg, and vanilla extract. Mix until well combined.

3 Fill the wells of a standard 12-cup muffin tin about halfway with the batter.

4 Bake in the preheated oven for 25 minutes.

5 Set the pan on a wire rack to cool completely before serving.

VARIATION TIP: Add a dollop of peanut butter or Cream Cheese Icing (page 22) to take these up a notch.

PER SERVING (1 BROWNIE)

Macronutrients: Fat 79%; Protein 7%; Carbs 14%
Calories: 288; Total Fat: 24g; Protein: 5g;
Total Carbs: 13g; Fiber: 8g; Net Carbs: 5g;
Erythritol 20g

LEMON SQUARES

— MAKES 9 SQUARES —

Tart Lemon Squares are a great summer dessert. And don't tell anyone, but I also love to eat them for breakfast with a cup of hot coffee. It may sound crazy, but it works, because really any time of day is the best time of day to eat Lemon Squares.

PREP TIME: 10 MINUTES

COOK TIME: 50 MINUTES

– 5 INGREDIENTS

6 tablespoons coconut oil, melted (olive oil works fine here, too), plus more for greasing the baking dish

1 lemon, quartered and seeded

4 large eggs

1 cup Swerve granular (or other granulated alternative sweetener)

1 Preheat the oven to 325°F. Grease a 9-inch square baking dish.

2 Put the lemon wedges (including the peel) in the blender and add the eggs, sweetener, and oil. Blend until smooth.

3 Pour the mixture into the prepared baking dish and bake for 50 minutes, or until set. Cool on a rack before cutting into squares to serve.

INGREDIENT TIP: For a beautiful dessert plate, serve these topped with dairy-free whipped cream and a few blueberries.

PER SERVING (1 SQUARE)

Macronutrients: Fat 86%; Protein 10%; Carbs 4%
Calories: 115; Total Fat: 11g; Protein: 3g; Total Carbs: 2g; Fiber: 0g; Net Carbs: 2g; Erythritol 20g

PUMPKIN CHEESECAKE

— SERVES 10 —

Cheesecake without the cream cheese (or any other dairy)! This Pumpkin Cheesecake is perfect for autumn and, of course, makes a great holiday-season dessert. You can make these in a muffin tin for mini cheesecakes, or cook up one full-size cake.

PREP TIME: 20 MINUTES
COOK TIME: 1 HOUR

6 tablespoons coconut oil, plus more for greasing the pan

1 cup almonds

1 (8-ounce) container dairy-free cream cheese (such as Kite Hill), at room temperature

4 large eggs

½ cup Swerve granular (or other granulated alternative sweetener)

½ cup pure pumpkin purée

2 teaspoons vanilla extract

1½ teaspoons ground cinnamon

1 teaspoon ground allspice

1 teaspoon ground ginger

1 teaspoon ground cloves

1 Preheat the oven to 350°F. Grease a standard 12-cup muffin tin or a 9-inch pie plate with coconut oil.

2 In a blender or food processor, combine the coconut oil and almonds, and process until finely ground.

3 Press the almond mixture into the bottom of the prepared muffin tin or pie plate, and refrigerate while you make the filling.

4 In a large mixing bowl, combine the cream cheese, eggs, sweetener, pumpkin purée, vanilla extract, cinnamon, allspice, ginger, and cloves, and beat to mix well.

5 Remove the chilled crust from the refrigerator and pour in the filling mixture.

6 Bake in the preheated oven for 1 hour, or until the center is set.

INGREDIENT TIP: You can use any oil here. When I have it on hand, I like to use walnut oil in place of the coconut oil because the flavor goes so well with pumpkin.

PER SERVING
Macronutrients: Fat 80%; Protein 11%; Carbs 9%
Calories: 246; Total Fat: 22g; Protein: 7g; Total
Carbs: 5g; Fiber: 2g; Net Carbs: 3g; Erythritol 10g

CHOCOLATE CHIP SKILLET COOKIE

— SERVES 4 —

This is such an easy dessert to throw together when you need something sweet. I love putting it in the oven as we sit down to eat—then, once dinner is finished and the kitchen is clean, we have dessert all ready to go. Throw some coconut whipped cream or dairy-free ice cream on top for an extra-special treat.

PREP TIME: 10 MINUTES

COOK TIME: 25 MINUTES

– 5 INGREDIENTS

Coconut oil, for greasing the skillet

1 cup low-carb baking mix (I like Bob's Red Mill)

¾ cup Swerve granular (or other granulated alternative sweetener)

¾ cup cacao butter, melted

2 teaspoons vanilla extract

¼ cup dairy-free chocolate chips

1 Preheat the oven to 350°F. Grease a 7-inch cast iron skillet with coconut oil.

2 In a mixing bowl, stir together the low-carb baking mix and sweetener. Add the melted cacao butter and vanilla extract, and mix until well combined. Fold in the chocolate chips.

3 Pour the mixture into the greased skillet and bake for 25 minutes

VARIATION TIP: Add ¼ cup chopped walnuts or pecans and ¼ cup shredded coconut to the mix for an amped-up version.

PER SERVING

Macronutrients: Fat 93%; Protein 3%; Carbs 4%
Calories: 415; Total Fat: 43g; Protein: 3g; Total Carbs: 4g; Fiber: 1g; Net Carbs: 3g; Erythritol 36g

CHOCOLATE BACON WITH PINK HIMALAYAN SALT

— SERVES 10 —

In case you thought keto was boring, I bring you salted-chocolate bacon. Be warned: You *will* want to eat all of these at one time. Try to resist. Try to share with your loved ones. Try.

PREP TIME: 10 MINUTES (PLUS 2 HOURS FOR FREEZING)

– ONE POT

– NO COOK

– 5 INGREDIENTS

1 batch Perfect Bacon (page 31), cooled

½ batch Chocolate Sauce (page 23)

1 tablespoon pink Himalayan salt

1 Arrange the bacon on a large rimmed baking sheet and drizzle the chocolate sauce over the top.

2 Sprinkle with the salt and freeze for at least 2 hours, or until hardened.

3 Serve chilled or store in a zip-top bag in the freezer for up to 3 months. (Who are we kidding? It'll be gone long before that.)

VARIATION TIP: Break each piece of bacon in half for bite-size pieces, and add one pecan to each piece while the chocolate is still runny. I love making these to bring to a holiday party.

PER SERVING

Macronutrients: Fat 82%; Protein 15%; Carbs 3%
Calories: 264; Total Fat: 24g; Protein: 10g; Total Carbs: 2g; Fiber: 0g; Net Carbs: 2g

CHOCOLATE CHIP PIE

— SERVES 10 —

When I made this pie for the first time, I ended up making it three more times that week. It cooks beautifully and tastes even better. Note that when the pie comes out of the oven, it will appear not to be fully cooked. Resist the urge to cook it longer, as it will become overbaked. Instead, refrigerate it until completely set.

PREP TIME: 20 MINUTES

COOK TIME: 40 MINUTES (PLUS 2 HOURS FOR CHILLING)

– 5 INGREDIENTS

FOR THE CRUST

2 cups almonds

1 cup cacao butter, melted

FOR THE FILLING

4 large eggs

¾ cup cacao butter, melted

¾ cup Swerve granular (or other granulated alternative sweetener)

½ cup dairy-free chocolate chips

TO MAKE THE CRUST

1 Preheat the oven to 350°F.

2 In a blender, blend the almonds and melted cacao butter. Spread the mixture out in a 9-inch pie plate. Using wet fingers, press the mixture down to spread it and smooth it out.

3 Bake in the preheated oven for 10 minutes.

4 Remove from the oven (but leave the oven on), and chill in the refrigerator while you make the filling.

TO MAKE THE FILLING

1 In a mixing bowl, combine the eggs, cacao butter, and sweetener. Stir in the chocolate chips.

2 Pour the batter into the chilled crust and bake for 30 minutes.

3 Chill until set, at least 2 hours, and serve cold.

SUBSTITUTION TIP: For a coconut cream pie, replace the chocolate chips with shredded coconut and top with coconut whipped cream.

PER SERVING

Macronutrients: Fat 90%; Protein 5%; Carbs 5%
Calories: 538; Total Fat: 54g; Protein: 7g; Total Carbs: 6g; Fiber: 4g; Net Carbs: 2g; Erythritol 14g

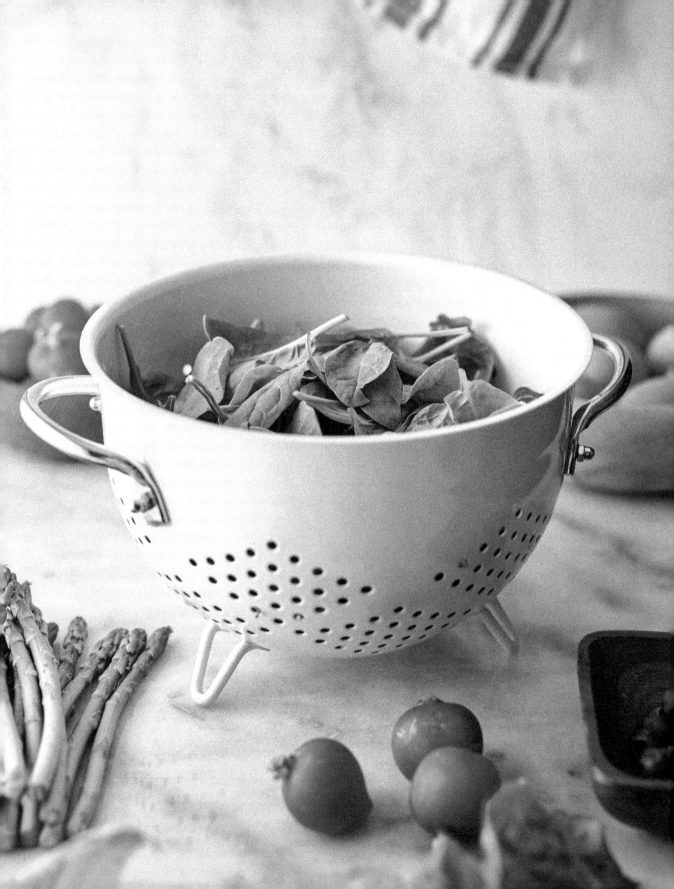

THE DIRTY DOZEN & THE CLEAN FIFTEEN™

A nonprofit environmental watchdog organization called Environmental Working Group (EWG) looks at data supplied by the U.S. Department of Agriculture (USDA) and the Food and Drug Administration (FDA) about pesticide residues. Each year it compiles a list of the best and worst pesticide loads found in commercial crops. You can use these lists to decide which fruits and vegetables to buy organic to minimize your exposure to pesticides and which produce is considered safe enough to buy conventionally. This does not mean they are pesticide-free, though, so wash these fruits and vegetables thoroughly.

Dirty Dozen™

- apples
- celery
- cherries
- grapes
- nectarines
- peaches
- pears
- potatoes
- spinach
- strawberries
- sweet bell peppers
- tomatoes

Additionally, nearly three-quarters of hot pepper samples contained pesticide residues

Clean Fifteen™

- asparagus
- avocados
- broccoli
- cabbages
- cantaloupes
- cauliflower
- eggplants
- honeydew melons
- kiwis
- mangoes
- onions
- papayas
- pineapples
- sweet corn
- sweet peas (frozen)

MEASUREMENT CONVERSIONS

Volume Equivalents (Liquid)

STANDARD	US STANDARD (OUNCES)	METRIC (APPROXIMATE)
2 tablespoons	1 fl. oz.	30 mL
¼ cup	2 fl. oz.	60 mL
½ cup	4 fl. oz.	120 mL
1 cup	8 fl. oz.	240 mL
1½ cups	12 fl. oz.	355 mL
2 cups or 1 pint	16 fl. oz.	475 mL
4 cups or 1 quart	32 fl. oz.	1 L
1 gallon	128 fl. oz.	4 L

Oven Temperatures

FAHRENHEIT (F)	CELSIUS (C) (APPROXIMATE)
250°	120°
300°	150°
325°	165°
350°	180°
375°	190°
400°	200°
425°	220°
450°	230°

Volume Equivalents (Dry)

STANDARD	METRIC (APPROXIMATE)
⅛ teaspoon	0.5 mL
¼ teaspoon	1 mL
½ teaspoon	2 mL
¾ teaspoon	4 mL
1 teaspoon	5 mL
1 tablespoon	15 mL
¼ cup	59 mL
⅓ cup	79 mL
½ cup	118 mL
⅔ cup	156 mL
¾ cup	177 mL
1 cup	235 mL
2 cups or 1 pint	475 mL
3 cups	700 mL
4 cups or 1 quart	1 L

Weight Equivalents

STANDARD	METRIC (APPROXIMATE)
½ ounce	15 g
1 ounce	30 g
2 ounces	60 g
4 ounces	115 g
8 ounces	225 g
12 ounces	340 g
16 ounces or 1 pound	455 g

RESOURCES

PeaceLoveAndLowCarb.com

Kyndra Holley is a genius at developing recipes and providing resources for the low-carb community. Her books boast beautiful insights and recipes for living the keto life. Instagram: @PeaceLoveAndLowCarb

KetoKarma.com

Suzanne Ryan is the first person I started to follow when I was learning about keto. Her website has always been my go-to when anyone has asked me hard questions that I need help answering. Her book *Simply Keto* is also lovely. Instagram: @KetoKarma

TheCastawayKitchen.com

Cristina Curp is a such a gift to anyone interested in clean eating and learning how to make your body work optimally for you. Her book *Made Whole* is a masterpiece. Instagram: @TheCastawayKitchen

Whole30.com

Doing a round of Whole30 is what introduced me to my dairy-free keto life. It taught me about my body and how living without dairy is doable and sustainable. Instagram: @Whole30

HealthfulPursuit.com

Leanne Vogel is a rock star when it comes to the keto diet. I love watching her learn, grow, and then impart her wisdom to the keto community. Instagram: @HealthfulPursuit

REFERENCES

HARVARD T.H. CHAN PUBLIC SCHOOL OF HEALTH. "The Microbiome." The Nutrition Source. Accessed September 12, 2018. https://www.hsph.harvard.edu/nutritionsource /microbiome/.

NATIONAL INSTITUTES OF HEALTH. "Lactose Intolerance." Genetics Home Reference. Accessed September 15, 2018. https://ghr.nlm.nih.gov/condition /lactose-intolerance#statistics.

U.S. DEPARTMENT OF HEALTH AND HUMAN SERVICES, HEALTH RESOURCES AND SERVICES ADMINISTRATION, MATERNAL AND CHILD HEALTH BUREAU. "Endocrine and Metabolic Disorders." *Women's Health USA 2009.* Accessed September 15, 2018. https://mchb.hrsa.gov/whusa09/hstat/hi/pages/217emd.html.

RECIPE INDEX

INDEX

ACKNOWLEDGMENTS

Brad, I love you. Thank you for being my constant cheerleader in life and through the process of writing this book. Thank you for keeping the kitchen clean when I was creating recipes and making emergency trips to the grocery store when I forgot key ingredients. You are the very best. I did it! We did it!

Thanks to Peggy and Vern, our poodles; I wrote much of this cookbook from 5:00 to 8:00 every morning, holding Vern in my lap, with Peggy right by my side.

Mom, thank you for teaching me how to cook. I learned how to love people well merely by observing you. I love you.

Kristen and Kate, thank you for coming through in the clutch in Arizona!

Lori, Bessie, and Mik, y'all are my people. Thank you for the gift of true friendship.

Brooke, thank you for always being all-in with everything I do.

Syd and Christina, thank you for always saying yes.

My team at Callisto Media, thank you. Pippa and Bridget, thank you for taking my words and making them more beautiful.

To my readers and my Instagram community, thank you for everything you have given me. I am so thankful to be able to write this book for you.

And to the Creator of the Stars, thank you for blessing me. I promise to continue using my talents to the best of my abilities.

ABOUT THE AUTHOR

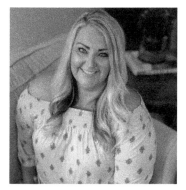

Jessica Dukes is a motivator and the founder of DailyKetosis.org. She loves to cook, create, and inspire others to live happier, healthier lives on her Instagram page, @DailyKetosis. Jessica lives in Nashville, Tennessee, with her husband, Brad, and their two poodles, Peggy and Vern.

CPSIA information can be obtained
at www.ICGtesting.com
Printed in the USA
BVHW091355091118
532664BV00021B/877/P